DLC—1,000+

(Delicious Low Cholesterol—1,000 Calories or More)

DLC–1,000+

(Delicious Low Cholesterol–1,000 Calories or More)

Defeat the Barriers to Healthful Eating.

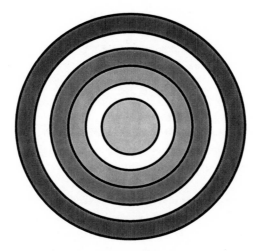

**Enjoy Living in the Jungle of
Delicious Food Products and Modern Services.**

Shrikant Bembalkar, MD

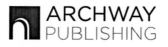

Archway Publishing books may be ordered through booksellers or by contacting:

Archway Publishing
1663 Liberty Drive
Bloomington, IN 47403
www.archwaypublishing.com
1-(888)-242-5904

Authors Note to readers:
This book expresses the opinions and ideas of its author. It is intended to provide
interesting and useful information in general and not specific individual diagnosis
or treatment. There is no intention to diagnose or to treat any specific individual.

Because of the dynamic nature of the Internet, any web addresses or
links contained in this book may have changed since publication and
may no longer be valid. The views expressed in this work are solely those
of the author and do not necessarily reflect the views of the publisher,
and the publisher hereby disclaims any responsibility for them.

Any people depicted in stock imagery provided by Thinkstock are models,
and such images are being used for illustrative purposes only.
Certain stock imagery © Thinkstock.

ISBN: 978-1-4808-0850-8 (sc)
ISBN: 978-1-4808-0851-5 (e)

Library of Congress Control Number: 2014910648

Printed in the United States of America.

Archway Publishing rev. date: 7/31/2014

To the mirror, who keeps me on track

If you know the enemy and yourself, you need not fear the results of one hundred battles.

If you know yourself but not the enemy, for every victory gained you will also suffer a defeat.

If you know neither the enemy nor yourself, you will succumb in every battle.

—SUN TZU

Contents

Preface

All of us want to eat right, enjoy what we eat, and stay healthy. Some of us have limited time; some of us have limited skills; some of us have limited information. Some of us have lots of our own "special" barriers.

Do you want to know how to defeat these barriers and eat delicious, healthy meals for the rest of your life?

This book is about overcoming these barriers to healthful eating. This book is not a textbook of nutrition or cooking. Based on more than forty years of experience in clinical medical practice, I have written this book to show how to overcome barriers that prevent people from eating healthfully.

In this book, in his own words, George describes to his dinner guests, including myself, the story of his struggles, setbacks, and success in developing healthful eating habits. The style is conversational, with very simple dialogues. Individuals tell their stories and ask their simple questions. I relate George's story while adding my own additional thoughts about the barriers to healthful eating.

George and his friends show you how they encountered and defeated the barriers and developed their own simple NEET (nutrition, ease, environment, taste) style (DLC 1,000+), suitable for any individual's taste, skills, and budget.

In his younger days, George ate with his mother's guidance and her concern about his nutrition. Later in life, for many reasons, George changed his emphasis from nutrition to taste and convenience. Gradually his eyes opened. With the help of information sources and modern products and services, George learned new methods and changed his emphasis toward nutrition, without compromising taste and convenience. Instead of blaming the new products and services, George learned to use modern products and services to his advantage.

Modifying pleasurable, long-standing habits is not an easy task. No one can tell what will motivate each one of you to change, but you will find plenty of stories in this book that will help you find the answers that, I hope, will work for you.

Sincerely,
S. L. Bembalkar, MD

Acknowledgments

Thanks to my mom, who showed me that it was easy to cook.

Thanks to my dad, who instilled in me the value of learning and questioning.

Thanks to my family and friends who have enjoyed my cooking and helped me learn a great deal more along the way.

Thanks also to AccessHealth for the infrastructure and colleagues at work for their support.

Thanks to Carroll and Wanda Simpkins for their valuable suggestions and encouragement.

Thanks to the many teachers, professors, speakers, newspapers, journals, magazines, and TV talk shows that helped me understand the complexities of this issue.

Special thanks to Mr. Gireesh Bembalkar for his penetrating questions and comments that helped me acquire a special insight regarding the barriers to healthful eating.

Thanks also to Archway Publishing for making it all possible.

Introduction

The Enemy = the Army of Barriers

"Good morning. How are you today, Mrs. Johnson?" asked the nurse.

"Just fine, thank you," replied Mrs. Johnson politely.

She had said it as a reflex, but underneath she was not so sure. She knew that she had not been able to show any improvement in her weight. She had tried her best, and yet the scales were going against her. "How is it possible?" she murmured to herself. She was hungry all the time. She had said no to her favorite pecan pie on Christmas Eve. She knew she could eat more. Her stomach growled almost every time she left the table. And yet the scales could not be wrong. She wanted to ask the nurse, "Is it possible to eat smaller quantities of food and still not be able to lose weight?"

"Congratulations, George. You have done it—and in spite of the holiday season," someone was heard saying. As George came out of the doctor's office with a bright smile on his face, everyone in the waiting room had eyes fixed on him. Everyone present had the same questions for George. "How did you do it, George? What is your secret?"

Ann had tears in her eyes. She knew she was overweight. She had tried her best. She had read magazines, attended programs, and tried special diets, but nothing had worked for her for long. She was sad, frustrated, and angry, and she wanted to know why.

Benjamin had been scared stiff about his cholesterol and his weight since he had learned recently about his neighbor's stroke at age fifty-two. He wanted to do something about his diet but did not know how.

Catherine was anxious. She was a traveling salesperson. She had no time to be picky about her diet. She had to eat on the run. She was ambitious. She enjoyed power lunches. She wanted to know what and where to eat.

Doris wanted to know when she should start being concerned about the diet of her family. They were young and healthy, and she wanted them to stay that way.

Edward was wondering about the articles in the newspaper and programs on TV and radio about the incidence of heart disease, colon cancer, and diabetes and their connection with diet factors. He wondered whether it was true or only media hype. His family was raised on the farm, and he just was not sure whether he needed to change anything.

Farrah had just moved away from her home in West Virginia to her own apartment in Chicago and had never really cooked a whole meal.

You have no doubt met Ann, Benjamin, Catherine, Doris, and many others who face barriers to healthful eating. In this book, George and his friends show you how they encountered and defeated the barriers and developed their own simple, NEET (nutrition, ease, environment, taste) style (DLC 1,000+) suitable for any individual's taste, skills, and budget.

So what are *your* barriers? Are *you* ready to fight the enemy?

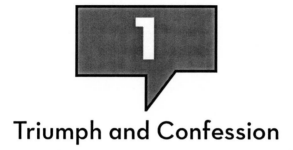

Triumph and Confession

A journey of a thousand miles begins with a single step.
—JAPANESE PROVERB

" **H**ow did you do it, George? Will you tell us the secret of your success?" Debra asked. Debra was a mother of three. She had read many recipe books but soon realized that one or two recipes don't make the entire day's eating. She tried to read all the food labels, but how much time could she spend reading labels? Reading books had not helped her much yet. Debra was waiting to ask someone like George about his secret formula.

The spacious waiting room in the New Way Clinic was crowded with people. It was a beautiful, sunny afternoon. The sun was shining brightly through the skylights, which made it easy to see the stress on everyone's face. Earlier today, George had also been there in the waiting room. He had just turned forty. He was there to get a routine physical. Benjamin, Justin, James, Helen, and I were also in the waiting room that afternoon and knew George. George had been in private practice with this group of physicians for many years at a different location. When George had been waiting for his visit with the doctor, he too had appeared a little nervous, but now, as he was walking out of the exam room, he was smiling again.

It was obvious that George had been quite successful in controlling the middle-age spread around the waist. It was also noticeable that he had gotten a good report overall. So when he came out smiling, he was bombarded with questions and nervous smiles from almost everyone in the waiting room.

"George, how did you do it? Will you tell us the secret of your success?" inquired Benjamin loudly, so that everyone could hear.

George answered, "Ben, do you really want me to bore you with another long lecture?"

Benjamin, Justin, James, Helen, and I were speechless. We did not know how to respond to that. We certainly did not want another lecture—neither long nor short, neither deeply scientific nor interesting. No lectures. There was complete silence.

"Would you mind showing us just how you did it and sharing with us your experience?" murmured Justin.

"I will be glad to share with you the story of my success. How shall we do it?" asked George. Then he paused for a minute and said, "I have an idea. Why don't you come on over for dinner tonight and be sure to invite Richard and Edward, also." Then George turned to Justin and asked, "Justin, how do you like your food? Do you like it hot and spicy, sour, not so spicy, sweet and sour?" George then asked Benjamin, "Ben, is there something you're allergic to?" Finally, George asked Helen, "Helen, is there something that you don't like? This last category is just to see whether I can fix it in such a way that you don't dislike it anymore."

Benjamin and I were simply shocked at his boldness and confidence. All of us knew that George had not cooked at all a couple of years ago.

Helen thought it was unlike George to be so boastful—to accept so many restrictions and challenges on such short notice! How could he do it in such a short time with such confidence?

Promptly at 7:00 p.m., all of us showed up at his house, as George had requested.

George was all dressed up and was comfortably watching the evening news on TV. "How can he be all done with his cooking? He must have ordered a pizza," Benjamin said, his curiosity boiling over. Although there was no aroma of a supreme pizza, Benjamin checked out his kitchen anyway. The kitchen was just an ordinary kitchen with ordinary kitchen appliances. The work table had some pots and pans on it, but they were covered. The dining table was nicely decorated and set with regular tableware. "Oh, sure, a TV dinner of some sort," remarked Justin.

"Dinner is ready," George announced.

After the initial pleasantries, we were seated at the dining table, and he served us a steaming hot dinner. His menu included bread, rice, lentil soup, two different vegetable dishes, two different salads, condiments, and a dessert. At first, when George said that he was not going to join us for the dinner and would like to eat later, Richard became skeptical about the whole affair.

"Why not? What's wrong? Are you afraid of something?" Richard asked.

The food looked okay. The aroma was different, but it was certainly appetizing. George said he was somewhat anxious, but he did not look a bit anxious to us. When Justin asked George about this, George said, "I don't know whether there will be enough, and I may have to fix something quick." George was not joking this time. When the initial apprehension was gone, Justin was secretly glad after the first bite that he had George's portion of the meal too.

The dinner was a complete success. All the plates were licked clean, and even the pots were almost empty.

"How did you do it, George? All of us want to know all the details—the whole story. We want to be able to do what you have done," Benjamin insisted.

As we were having coffee right after dinner, George looked at us and confessed, "As all of you know, it was not exactly like this, even just a few years ago."

"We know that; one year ago you couldn't cook, except maybe for yourself," said James almost sarcastically.

"You're right," agreed George. "One year ago, I didn't have many things. I did not have the skill. I felt that it was not a man's job to cook. I thought that it was not necessary for a man to be in the kitchen unless he was trying to be a professional chef. Mind you, I accepted the idea that men can be great cooks if they like that type of work or if they have to do it for a livelihood, but I was a doctor. I could not be a cook, neither a great one nor an ordinary one. I didn't have the time to learn to cook even if I wanted to. I didn't have the time to cook even if I learned it. I could not be tied down for hours of tedious manual labor. I felt I had other important things to do."

"Besides, it wasn't necessary. What are wives for, anyway?" came the smart-aleck comment from Richard.

"And if there is no wife, then there was the dinner in the hospital cafeteria or any of the fine restaurants in the area," Edward noted.

"I didn't even know the basics—ingredients, measurements, or even the process of cooking." George was trying to give all the reasons that he could list.

"Did your mom not teach you anything?" James interrupted.

"My mother taught me many things when I was a kid. I had to help her with the chores in the kitchen almost every day. Over the years, I forgot the information and lost the skills. Of course, the library had many books, the stores in the mall were full of interesting books on this subject, and the Internet had a vast collection of material on this subject as well. The TV had programs, and the local hospital had classes. But I just didn't have the time *or* the interest. I didn't care. It didn't matter," George said almost apologetically and added that Kroger, McDonald's, Taco Bell, the Char, and many other places were always there, with friendly service. They were ready day and night, here, there, and everywhere around the world, and sometimes just at the end of the telephone or a quick message on the smartphone.

"And all of them have many delicious items to offer at a very reasonable price and great speed," Edward pointed out.

"Oh, yes. I agree completely. As a matter of fact, I liked to eat out for a number of reasons. My main reason was that I hated the chores in the kitchen," said George as his final excuse.

All of us dinner guests agreed with him every step of the way, especially regarding his final excuse.

"What happened then? What changed you? How did you do it, George?" Catherine blurted out loudly. Her anxiety was obvious.

"And then something happened," George confessed in a monotone.

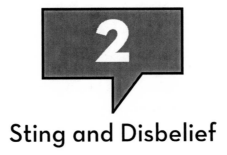

Sting and Disbelief

Negligence is a powerful enemy.

—EDWIN HOYT

George pulled up a chair and sat down. All of a sudden he became serious and said, "It usually takes four stings for me to change. One to wake up. One more to feel the pain. One more to come to my senses. One more to start action to change.

"In this particular situation, to learn to cook and eat right, it took a whole lot more stings. I experienced innumerable stings before I moved from one category to the next. And all of that took a long time.

"For years we have been told that 'you are what you eat.' We are told that diet has a lot to do with our health and disease, but we ignore it, and I was no exception. Let me tell you what happened to me on my thirty-fifth birthday. Just like today, I was in the clinic getting my annual checkup. I was feeling well, and I didn't have any symptoms to discuss. So I was quite surprised after the checkup.

"'What are you doing to yourself, George? It seems that the good life has been catching up with you,' Dr. John said to me with a tap on my shoulder.

"I didn't understand. I thought John was complimenting me. I smiled and was about to tell John about my new car, the trip my wife and I had taken to the beach, and the delicious foods we enjoyed in different restaurants.

"'Didn't you buy a new refrigerator last year? That model must be user friendly. You've put on more than twenty pounds on your belly; your cholesterol level is certainly not what it should be. You need to work on that,' Dr. John said in his plain, clear, and quite blunt style.

"I still didn't fully understand the implications of what John had just said, and as soon as I walked out of the doctor's office I forgot about the whole episode.

"A month or so later, one evening my wife and I were walking around in the mall after our dinner at the New China restaurant. We'd had a very good dinner, and we were walking slowly, browsing here and there, when my wife noticed that there was a long line of people waiting in front of a small booth. It was Healthscreen, a program conducted by one of the local hospitals. On that particular day, they were doing cholesterol tests. Not surprisingly, my wife insisted that I should get my cholesterol rechecked. Naturally, I was not interested.

"'Why not? It's free,' said someone who was waiting in line. 'Why not?' said I, and I joined the line. The technician was very good. To get the drop of blood for the test, she stuck the ring finger in my left hand with a sharp lancet. It didn't hurt much. She asked me to wait a little while longer and then gave me the report. 'Two thirty-nine. Your test result is abnormal,' the technician said to me and added, 'Please see your doctor soon; you may want to repeat the test.'"

"Along with the test result, I received some brochures and informational materials. I couldn't read the materials there in the mall, and I didn't want to carry those papers with me, so I found an excuse. 'My arm is beginning to hurt, and I can't carry these papers with me,' I said. Before my wife could find a simple solution, the materials were in the garbage can, and we were on our way to the movie theater. My wife was concerned about the number. My reaction was different. I didn't want to believe the number. I was doubtful about the little, unsophisticated machine and its accuracy. 'Probably a laboratory error,' I told myself. 'Or it could be because of the big dinner I had. Technical error. Nothing is bothering me.' That is how I reacted. Then we went to see a movie. The movie was very good. It was a high-tech thriller. The hero won every time in spite of all the dangers from the evil forces! By the time we finished watching the movie, the memory of the abnormal test was already fading away fast.

"Within a few days I had forgotten about the whole thing, but then my telephone rang in the middle of the night. That itself was not so unusual for me. I picked up the phone. John, who had been my classmate in high school, was at the other end. His voice was hoarse as if he had been crying. 'Have you heard the bad news?' John asked. 'No. What is it?' I asked. 'Our friend Jeremy passed away suddenly, earlier today at his home of a massive heart attack,' John informed me.

"I was stunned. Jeremy was a little younger than I. He must have been about thirty-two years old. Jeremy was married and had two small children. John and I talked a little longer, and when I hung up the telephone I had a very deep, heavy, sinking feeling in my heart. I tried to sleep but couldn't. My mind was overrun with questions, thoughts, and memories of Jeremy.

"'Why? What could be the reason? Could it have been prevented? He was a little overweight and had a mild high-blood-pressure problem. He was on a small amount of medications. He may have had diabetes. He smoked cigarettes, but only occasionally. He probably had family history. **That** is why this must have happened. It's not going to happen to me. I don't smoke, I don't feel bad, I have no hypertension, and my grandfather lived to be ninety years old. No need to worry,' I said to myself.

"A week after that telephone call I attended a dinner and continuing medical education program at the country club. The ambiance was pleasant as usual. Beautiful décor, soft music, light conversation, relaxed atmosphere. I had already forgotten about the blood tests, but Jeremy's passing was still haunting me. I was hungry after a busy day. The chef had done his best again. The program started after the dinner was served. Rose, the coordinator of the program, announced the speaker and the topic. When I heard what she said, the steak knife almost fell out of my hand. You guessed it right. The speaker was a well-known professor from a reputable university, but the topic wasn't exactly what I wanted to hear about. He was going to talk about heart disease, obesity, and diet.

"I heard everything the speaker said that evening and disagreed with everything. I disagreed for no particular good reason. I just disagreed. And whatever I couldn't disagree with, I forgot quickly and conveniently. You may not believe it, but the next day, I didn't even remember that I went to the meeting at all. I didn't want to believe it. I was happy the way I was. I didn't want to change anything.

"I didn't want to change my lifestyle, especially my eating habits. Subconsciously, I probably knew that if I agreed with the speaker and remembered what he said, I would have to change.

"The next day I woke up feeling a little uneasy. I wasn't tired. I had had a good sleep. But I was uneasy, and I didn't know why. I wasn't even sure whether I wanted to find out why I was feeling that way. I just wanted to pull the blinds over my eyes and pretend that nothing had ever happened that a double-cheese pizza with several special toppings later that day for lunch couldn't cure.

"I blamed the uneasy feeling on a bad dream I didn't have, bad back I didn't have, and a soft new bed which also I did not have. I guess I just wanted to blame something for what was happening."

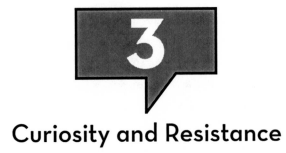

Curiosity and Resistance

There is no medicine to cure a fool.

—ANONYMOUS

"Tell me, George, did the pizza help?" asked Cathy, who was always on the road due to her job as a salesperson.

"No. It did not help at all to get rid of the uneasy feeling, but something else happened at lunch that made me feel a little better," George answered with a smile.

"What was that?" asked Cathy.

"John invited me to come over for dinner at his home."

"What is so special about that?"

George smiled again and said, "I have been to John's home for dinner many times, but the dinner event that evening became special. The dinner itself at John's home was simple. No great decorations, no great formalities. There was pita bread, two vegetables, a salad, bean soup, rice, and a dessert. It was delicious. It was different. I ate well and enjoyed every morsel of it. His lovely wife, a gracious host, pushed me into taking second and third helpings. During the dinner, John described with great excitement his recent triumphs in tennis, current world affairs, and new computer games.

"Ordinarily, I would have been interested in everything John had to say on any topic. John is a well-respected colleague and a very good friend, but on that day I wasn't interested in his stories about tennis or the latest computer games. My mind was occupied with thoughts about the dinner. I enjoyed the dinner very much. I was thinking, 'Hey, this is good food, and I wish I could eat like this every day. The professors were telling me that if I kept up with my old ways, I was headed for trouble. Here's an attractive alternative. Should I try it? Can I do it?'"

"I wasn't yet sure. I really didn't want to change, and how could I change even if I wanted to? Then my mind went into a high gear: I couldn't change. I didn't know anything. I was too old to change. I didn't have the time. I didn't believe 'them' professors. I didn't believe those drug companies, their research studies, and their slick little brochures.

"Even though I was thinking to myself, it must have been pretty loud thinking, because I heard John ask, 'George, are you willing to investigate and educate yourself?'

"The bug named curiosity must have bitten me hard that day, and so I said, 'Sure, why not?'

"Somehow, when I heard myself say that, all of a sudden the uneasiness that I had felt all day disappeared."

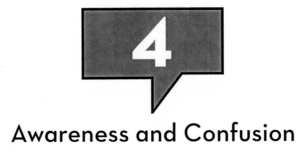

Awareness and Confusion

Shariram aadyam, khalu dharma-sadhanam.
Body (physical and mental health) is the first tool
to be able to perform duties of your daily life.
—SANSKRIT WORDS OF WISDOM

"How did that dinner change anything? And what is this bug named curiosity you are talking about? George, I don't want to be nosy, but you are making me very interested in this bug," Doris said anxiously.

"Very simple to answer that. This newfound curiosity sharpened my eyes and ears. I started to listen more carefully. I started to read with greater attention. I started to see what I did not see before. I began to see a different world. There was a revolution going on out there," George answered.

"The newspapers were filled with articles about diet and health," George continued. "The TV, the radio, the talk shows, and the magazines were all talking about the epidemic of obesity. One day, while I was walking around the hospital, I heard a young speaker talk excitedly in front of a charged audience of all ages, who were attending a patient-education class. I decided to join them. The speaker was saying, 'If we examine the eating habits of Americans, today we see a great change. From a society of hunters and gatherers, we have now become a society of consumers of processed food. During the past few years especially there has been a further substantial change in our approach to eating. Almost everyone nowadays prefers 'blue' milk to 'red' milk!'

"An older gentleman of about sixty or sixty-five years of age interrupted the speaker. 'Young man, will you please tell me what is this 'blue' milk and 'red' milk before we go on any further?' Interestingly, the fifteen-year-old grandson accompanying the older gentleman blurted out, 'The red milk is in the red box, and the blue milk is in the blue box. The regular and the 2 percent milk or the skim milk.' Everyone laughed.

"'You are absolutely correct, young man,' the speaker continued. 'These changes have been radical, profound, and on a very large scale, affecting the lives of millions of Americans—dramatic and rapid, almost like a revolution. I would like to call it the American Food Revolution. Why this revolution? Not because of an accident, an order by a dictator, or a fatwa by a religious leader, but because of the overwhelming consensus amongst researchers, scientists, government regulators, industry leaders, and the people themselves regarding the role of diet and nutrition in health, disease, and environmental matters. Scientists and researchers have given us new information regarding nutrition, health, food processing, and so on. Scientists have given us new technologies. Industry has certainly kept up with this and given us new products and new tools.' He went on and on and on.

"It was fascinating, especially his points about how things are changing in our information-driven society. I had heard it all before. I had seen it all before. I had known it all before.

"Somehow in the past it hadn't touched me or affected me the way it was affecting me on that day. In the past, I was like a water lily in the pond. Water drops didn't stick. I was in it and yet out of it. I was in the midst of it and yet completely oblivious to it. As I thought more, it became obvious to me. In different words and different diagrams and charts, all of these research studies were strongly pointing to the same conclusion, that diet is an important factor in the balance between health and disease, and these researchers had some solid recommendations regarding diet and nutrition.

"Here I was, perfectly happy with my own eating habits and lifestyle. I may have been a little overweight, and I may have had a little problem with the cholesterol blood test, but I enjoyed my food, and I didn't feel bad. Yet someone out there was telling me that I ought to change my direction.

"I wasn't yet so sure. I was irritated. I felt pressured by these professors and the blitz on the media. I enjoyed my food and my lifestyle; I didn't want anyone to tell me to change. I didn't want to give up on that just because someone said that I should.

"My mind was telling me one thing, and my brain was telling me something different. At that point, I decided to get out of the class. I decided that it was a good idea to go someplace quiet and peaceful, away from speeches, lectures, advice, orders, and the blitz in the media.

"I decided to go for a walk in the woods."

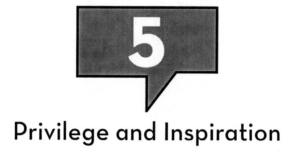

Privilege and Inspiration

When you arise in the morning, think of what a precious
privilege it is to be alive, to breathe, to think, to enjoy, to love.
—MARCUS AURELIUS

"So I went for a walk in Grandview Park with my friend John," George said. "I have learned that the gentle walking trails in these parks are the best medicine for the confused, irritated, disturbed, restless mind, and on that particular day that walk was the best medicine anyone could have had.

"It was a beautiful Saturday morning in the middle of the summer. Have you ever visited the parks in West Virginia? These are some of the most tranquil places in the whole world. I ought to know. I have traveled from one end of the world to the other.

"John and I hiked, examined the wildflowers, listened to the birds, and had a wonderful time. It was hard physical work at times, but it was exhilarating. The sight of the distant mountains, the sounds of the birds and the wind rustling through the leaves, the scent of the moist soil and the flowers, the feel of the gentle breeze, and the taste of the clear, cool water was absolutely fantastic. It is beyond my ability to describe the full impact on me on that day.

"I thanked the Lord for what he had bestowed upon me.

"John and I had known many who had disregarded and disrespected, knowingly or unknowingly, this *privilege*, this God-given gift of healthy life. Over the years, John and I had seen the suffering and misery these individuals had to face every day. Some could not walk without discomfort and pain; some could not breathe well; some could not swallow with ease and enjoy what they wanted to eat or drink. They could not enjoy the simplest activities that bring comfort and pleasure. They were in chronic misery of one kind or another, brought on mostly by their own unhealthy deeds.

"'How lucky can you get? Two legs, two arms, two eyes, two ears, a body, a mind, and a brain to appreciate and enjoy the beautiful world around me,' I said to myself. I felt privileged and deeply happy for all these God-given gifts, which many of us take for granted.

"One thing I was absolutely sure of at the end of my hike in the woods that day: I knew for certain that I wanted to respect and protect this privilege for as long as I could. At least, I didn't want to do something willfully that would diminish it or destroy it. "That was my inspiration to change," George said with peace, equanimity, and confidence.

"So, George, you made up your mind; found all good, acceptable reasons; did what you were supposed to do; and lived happily ever after. Is that what you are going to tell us next?" James asked sarcastically.

George almost completely ignored the biting comment and laughed. He remembered exactly how he felt the next day.

Reader Questions

What inspires you and motivates you? Why do you want to change your diet?

» *be proactive and pay attention to new information*

» *adjust diet to maintain a certain lifestyle*

» *do not want to disturb my golf game*

» *can go swimming*

» *do not want to spend a lot of money on health care*

» *do not want to be made fun of*

» *want to get a good job*

» *can get better styles of clothes*

» *make myself attractive to the opposite sex*

» *avoid skin infections like my grandmother*

» *avoid joint pains like my grandfather*

» *control my diabetes*

» *cut down on my medicines*

» *avoid preventable disease and dying early*

Magic Pill

When faced with a challenge, look for a way, not a way out.
—DAVID L. WEATHERFORD

"The next day, after a good night's sleep, my body was well rested, and my mind was fresh and ready to tackle any serious problems," George said. The irritation of the past few days was completely out of my mind. At breakfast in the hospital cafeteria as usual (a two-egg omelet, toast with butter and jam, sausage, some hash-brown potatoes, and a cup of coffee), John and I talked about the weekend. I told him about the wonderful day I'd had hiking with him in the woods and my thoughts about *the privilege.* John listened to me attentively and with interest.

"Then it was John's turn to tell me about his excellent tennis match in great detail. Usually I would have listened to him carefully and added my own comments, but I was still daydreaming about my day in Grandview Park and *the privilege*. It just wasn't possible for me to listen to what John was saying with interest and enthusiasm.

"'Wouldn't it be wonderful if there was a magic pill or a magic spell to keep us young and healthy forever?' I wondered aloud.

"John laughed heartily for a moment, showing his full set of glowing white teeth, and then suddenly he became very serious and said, 'George, I have a friend. He used to be my tennis partner for many years before you.'

"I knew immediately who John was talking about.

"'Jimmy was a great tennis player,' John continued, 'but he had a problem. Jimmy always thought that cigarettes wouldn't affect him the way they affected others. Nobody could convince him otherwise. So he smoked quite heavily. Eventually he had to slow down his tennis because of his breathing problems, and finally, last year, he had to quit playing tennis altogether. He couldn't enjoy it anymore with all that huffing and puffing.

"'You know also about my cousin Jerry. Great skier! The hamburger and hot dog man, who hated any kind of vegetables. 'Too bulky, too gassy,' he used to say. 'Cramps my style,' he used to grumble. Six months ago they told him that he has cancer of the colon.

"'And you must have heard about Steve. He liked to drive fancy, fast cars. He also liked to drink alcohol. He doesn't drive any cars at all anymore because his first and only accident has left him a paraplegic,' John continued.

"'Before they became incapacitated, all of them had told me how much they enjoyed living and doing what they were doing. Each one of them wanted a magic spell to stay young forever to play tennis, to ski, or to race fast cars. Now they know better, but it's too late for them to change anything that has already happened to them.

"'Don't you read the newspapers? Don't you hear the statistics on TV? Don't you know how many work hours are lost every day because of bad habits and their consequences?'

"John then turned his bright eyes straight on me and asked, 'Was it the magic pill that made you go through medical school when the others were enjoying the cinema, restaurants, and so on? Was it the magic pill that brought you to the USA? Is it the magic pill that makes you go to the woods to hike or makes you play tennis and exercise to keep yourself healthy and fit?'

"John continued, 'George, you had a goal, and you had to work hard to get there. You had to find out yourself what you wanted, and you had to go after it. You had to work hard to get it, and if you failed, you had to investigate your failure and then try again until you succeeded. No one else can do it for you. You have to do it yourself.'

"John took a deep breath, looked at me with his supportive, reassuring smile, and said, 'If the privilege of life and health is important to you, then look in the mirror and ask yourself, what are *you* willing to do to preserve it and protect it?'"

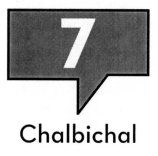

Chalbichal

One Step Forward, One Step Backward

There is no more miserable being than in whom nothing is habitual but indecision.

—WILLIAM JAMES

"John was not telling me anything new, nothing that I did not know before," George said. "I recognized that John wanted to let me know his strong feelings on this subject without belittling or ridiculing me in any way. He was making me face up to myself. John was making me ask myself some very difficult questions that I had avoided or ignored in the past: What do I really want? What am I going to do about it?

"I was stunned by his blunt, plain, simple words. Those questions gave me a lot to think about." George paused introspectively and added, "By the time John had finished talking to me that day, I had a lot more questions on my mind. I also knew that John was a perfect sounding board.

"'You like hiking, don't you?' I asked John.

"'Yes, of course,' John answered.

"'Would you like to go hiking with me this Saturday?'

"'Sure, why not, on any Saturday after my tennis game,' replied John.

"'Where and when shall we go?'

"'I enjoy hiking on comfortable terrain, more like walking on easy trails, and I would love to go for a walk on any such trail after a game of tennis,' John answered.

"'Could I ask you questions while we walk?'

"'Yes, of course, but I have one simple condition. For any new set of questions, we must find a new trail,' suggested John.

"That was not very difficult. There are many trails for a nice, easy walk in West Virginia. John and I decided to go on a new trail every Saturday morning, and to his surprise we needed all of those trails at least once, and some more than once, to present all my questions. As we were walking and talking one day about health, diet, and other things, John noticed the indecisiveness, doubts, and hesitation I had. He also noticed that I was becoming more and more uncomfortable about my questions on diet and health, a little embarrassed perhaps. One day John asked me, 'George, have you heard the story of the great warrior named Arjun and what happened to him just before the great war was about to begin?'

"'No. I don't remember very well, and what has Arjun the Great Archer to do with health, diet, and things like that anyway?' I shot back curtly. I knew that John had a tendency to tell stories instead of giving simple, straightforward answers. That was his way of explaining things or making a point. Sometimes it was okay. At other times it irritated me because I was looking for quick answers and quick, immediate solutions to my problems.

"'This way, *you* have to think and come to your own conclusions about whatever I'm saying,' John always said in his calm, confident voice when pushed to do otherwise.

"This was one of those occasions. I knew that John always had the best intentions for me. I felt I might have offended him with my last question, so I added quickly, 'But I'm willing to listen to the story of Arjun, if you think it's relevant. I promise I will listen with full attention.'

"John smiled and told me this story."

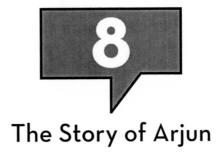

The Story of Arjun

Information, Knowledge, Doubts, and Wisdom

Doubt is a pain too lonely to know that Faith is his twin brother.
—KHALIL GIBRAN

" " " his story comes from the Mahabharata, a major Sanskrit epic of ancient India,' John began. 'Arjun was a great warrior prince. He had studied with the finest teachers and had mastered all the weapons of warfare. He had excelled in all the tests and situations. He was the greatest and most feared archer at that time.

"'Arjun's oldest brother, Dharma, was next in line for the throne. Unfortunately, Dharma was tricked into a gambling session by his rivals to the throne. Subsequently he lost his kingdom and all the wealth. He even lost personal freedom for himself, for his wife, and also for all his brothers, including the great archer Arjun. In addition, Dharma agreed to a condition that all of them had to leave the kingdom and live in exile for a period of thirteen years: twelve years anywhere in the jungles, outside the borders of their kingdom, and one year incognito. And if they were recognized during the thirteenth year or caught, they were to repeat the exile for thirteen more years!

"'During those thirteen years, these five princes and their queen had to suffer innumerable hardships and attempts on their lives. Their enemies tried their best many times to put them to death one way or another. Many times Arjun and his brothers almost lost their lives. After this period of hardships and danger for thirteen years, they returned safely and successfully. They expected to be treated with respect, honor, and love but were not treated fairly by their greedy cousins, who were ruling the kingdom. These five princes then made several attempts toward a peaceful settlement through negotiations. Finally, after all the peaceful attempts were exhausted, they decided to go to war and were facing each other's armies on the battlefield, all set to start a horrible war.

"'At this final moment, after all the information, preparations, deliberations, and decisions, Arjun the great warrior developed doubts about the usefulness of the war with his enemies. Arjun knew that a great warrior must not engage in the act of war on an impulse, even though he might be fully capable of winning that battle.

"'Arjun knew that, before engaging in any war, he must first clear all his doubts from his mind regarding the enemy and the need for war. This is the point I want to stress upon you.

"'Subsequently, of course, Arjun's doubts were removed after a lengthy question-and-answer session with his philosopher friend. After that the great warrior Arjun entered the war and won it in the end.'

"John finished telling me the story and asked, 'George, now you know how and why Arjun cleared his doubts. Now tell me what is really on your mind. What is bothering you? Why are you asking complicated, smart-sounding questions when it seems to me that you need answers to some very simple, basic questions?

"'Please feel free to ask any questions that will clear up your understanding of the subject. Please remember that no questions are silly questions. No questions are too small or insignificant. No doubts are too unimportant, especially if not raising them is stopping you from investigation and action.'"

Questions, Questions, Questions

Learn from yesterday, live for today, and hope for tomorrow. The important thing is not to stop questioning.

—ALBERT EINSTEIN

"So, George, did you really ask John simple, basic questions? Did that not bother you?" asked Ed guardedly.

"Yes. It did bother me at first. It was obvious. I was very uncomfortable about asking simple, basic questions because I was afraid that such questions would make me look stupid. With his straight talk, John had already made me feel a whole lot better, more at ease, and relaxed. After a few more minutes of walk on the trail, we decided that it was too late in the day for more questions. So we decided to keep more questions for the next trail.

"I was never afraid of asking questions except when I felt that a particular question would make me appear stupid in front of John. One of my favorite teachers from history is Socrates. The well-known

Greek philosopher is attributed with the saying, 'Unexamined life is not worth living.' Socrates had an interesting way of teaching. He taught by questioning his listeners. That is what fascinated me most.

"I had plenty of questions, and now I had a willing person, John, at whom to target them and his assurance that I would not be laughed at. Everyone has to eat every day, and there are so many choices. I started the fireworks:

> What should I eat?
>
> Why do I eat—for taste, nutrition, looks, or muscles?
>
> What is good for me?
>
> How much do I need?
>
> What about junk food, such as fast food, additives, preservatives, sweeteners, chewing gum, and cholesterol?
>
> What about food labels and health claims?
>
> What do I need to change?
>
> What about the environmental impact of what I do?
>
> What would my mother say?
>
> What does my doctor say?
>
> What are those professors saying? Why?
>
> Today, there is concern for nutrition as well as for taste. There is concern for the environment as well as for convenience. How do we take on this challenge?

"I would have gone on like this if John had not interrupted.

"'Whoa, whoa, whoa.' John stopped me. 'Not so fast, and not so many in a row. Simply speaking, what you're worried about is, How are we going to meet the challenge of better nutrition? How are we going to assure ourselves of quality nutrition in the jungle of products and services out there? What kind of diet do we need daily?' Then John smiled and said, 'Out of all your questions, let me choose the one most important question to tackle first. Let us choose this one: What would my mother say?'

"That question, John knew, was the perfect way for him to get out of being a crutch and instead to be a guide. My mother would have answered my questions by asking a question of her own. She would have asked, 'George, is what you are eating good for you?' Invariably, I would have answered, 'I don't know, but it sure tastes great,' which would have been followed immediately by her next question. 'George, don't you think you should find out first, before the damage is done? Go and find out yourself.'

"I could not escape the work of finding out, because 'George, what did you learn today? Please tell me all about it' used to be the next segment of our conversation.

"John knew all of this. So he added a few more of his own questions to my long list. 'George, how did you get here, to the USA? How did you gain so much weight? What are your goals? Objectives?'"

Looking Back

That men do not learn very much from the lessons of history is the most important of all the lessons of history.

—ALDOUS HUXLEY

Farrah had moved from West Virginia to Chicago. She knew how it felt to leave home and live away from family and close friends. She knew how many things changed. She asked George, "George, tell me, what do you remember about your travel to the New World?"

George answered, "I remember those days very well; as if it was only yesterday. I will describe to you my airplane travel in extra detail, as I remember it especially well.

"'What would you like to have for lunch, sir?' A very sweet and polite voice woke me from my light sleep. It was my first airplane trip. I was on my way to Colombo, Sri Lanka, to take a test to qualify for postgraduate medical training in the USA. The air hostess was passing out lunch boxes.

"I did not have an immediate answer to her question. I did not even know the choices. So I asked, 'What do you have?' She said something, but I did not quite understand the words. She had a different accent, and I know now that those words were not in my vocabulary at that time anyway. I don't remember how I answered, but soon I had a little plastic container in front of me. It contained a sandwich, some potato chips, and a pickled cucumber.

"I did not know anybody else on the airplane to ask any questions. I was hungry and nervous, so I opened the package and ate the sandwich. The sandwich tasted different than the coriander-and-potato sandwiches I was used to. It was bland and a little more salty, but it tasted alright. It wasn't enough to satisfy my appetite, so I asked for another one. It was of a different kind. I didn't ask what it contained, and there was no label on it telling me about its ingredients, calories, or fat grams. I assumed that the airline was a reputable company, everyone on the airplane was eating without getting sick, and it tasted okay and looked good. That was enough for me. Taste and appearance were the deciding factors.

"Looking back, however, I remember a neighboring passenger who had a very surprised look in his eyes. Now I know that he had good reason to be surprised. He knew, and I did not, that I was eating a ham-and-cheese sandwich. That, of course, was the beginning of a drastic change in my food choices. I didn't know it then, but I do know now. It was so subtle, so imperceptible, and yet so radical!

"In Colombo, along with bananas, mangoes, guavas, rice, dal, and everything else, I had a taste of an egg omelet fried in coconut oil. Everyone in the medical-college hostel where I was staying was enjoying his breakfast except me. I didn't like the taste at all, but I'm sure that, had I stayed in Colombo a little while longer, I would have developed a taste for it.

"I did well on my qualifying tests in Colombo, and several months later I was on my way to America for my postgraduate education.

"My connecting flight in Tehran could not wait for my delayed flight from Bombay, and I was bumped. The airline took care of all the passengers very well. They put us up in a large hotel with a nice restaurant. At dinner time, I came downstairs and was ushered in politely and seated at a table by myself. The waiter came and gave me a menu. It was printed in English, but the words were mostly unknown to me. A few minutes later the waiter reappeared.

"'How would you like your steak, sir?'

"I must have taken an unusually long time to answer, because before I could come up with an answer, he had disappeared. He returned a few minutes later, placed the dinner plate in front of me, waited politely for a few seconds to receive any further orders from me, and, when he noticed that none were coming, disappeared again.

"There wasn't much on the plate compared to the multiple vegetable dishes that I was used to. A brownish-black, square, thick lump; something green, a vegetable of some kind with golden-yellow sauce on it (I found out later that it was melted cheese); something soft and cream colored (mashed potatoes); a piece of bread; butter; and a bowl of tomato, cucumber, carrots, and something like a cabbage (salad). I was ready to eat. There was one problem, though. I had no idea what was on the plate and how to tackle it. I didn't want to make a fool of myself. I didn't want to call the waiter to ask him about the food and how to eat it. I was thinking, *With my hands? With my fork? Knife? Spoon? How do I mix it? What do I eat first?*

"I didn't have much of a choice in the matter of the menu. The people around me had the same type of food on their plates. I looked around to see how they were handling the food on their plates. I prayed once. When no answers came, I prayed again a few more times. Then, fortunately, the answer came. A passenger at the next table recognized that I had absolutely no idea how to eat the stuff in front of me. She was an English teacher from America. She smiled and showed me how to eat the American way. It was a surprise to me, but my stomach learned quickly to tackle any such difficulties with ease.

"My tongue also experienced a new challenge. During the next several years my tongue had the opportunity to experiment with an enormous variety of products from all over the world, in supermarkets, cafeterias, restaurants, and the homes of friends from different parts of the world. The daily routine was dictated by the working hours and the work environment. What I was going to eat was dictated by taste, convenience, and the mood of the moment. Mostly it was the tongue that was in charge of my eating now.

"My mother was happy with my photographs, which I sent to her with my letters. 'You must be a great cook by now. You have put on at least twenty pounds since you left home,' she wrote me once.

"She didn't know that I liked a double-egg omelet for my daily breakfast instead of the raw eggs that I had been forced to eat monthly as a kid. She had tried her best to make sure that I got enough nourishment. That is how the monthly routine of two raw eggs and a weekly spoonful of cod-liver oil got started. Those were the terror moments in my childhood.

"'Your health comes first,' my mother used to say.

"'No!' my tongue used to say every time I had to take the raw eggs or the spoonful of cod-liver oil, but my tongue never had the slightest chance of winning in that situation.

"In the past, my mother had looked after my nutrition the best way she knew how. When I was on my own, my tongue came to dominate my eating. I had changed completely and drastically. My mom emphasized my nutrition and the taste. When I was on my own, it was only the taste that decided what I ate. My mom was happy with my photographs; my tongue was happy with the omelets, hot dogs, and hamburgers; and I was happy because my mother was happy.

"Who was looking after my nutrition now? Nobody.

"It was crystal clear what John was pointing to. The professors, the government officials, the doctors, and in short the whole world were trying to change eating habits because of the new information that was available, and I had completely ignored the new information on nutrition. I was focused on the taste and convenience! I was going in a different direction than the rest of the educated world.

"Bang. Then it dawned on me.

"If I wanted to do something about my eating, I must first formulate my goals on paper."

Mission, Goals, Objectives

If you get the objectives right,
a lieutenant can write the strategy.
−GEN. GEORGE C. MARSHALL

George continued, "I went on a brainstorming spree for the next several weeks and came up with some great ideas, based on what I had learned from John:

Mission

To protect the privilege of health by putting into practice what the experts have known for a long time. At present, the emphasis has been on taste and convenience. In addition, one must also emphasize nutrition and environment (NEET).

Goals

Reduce risk factors in recipes and diet. Reduce salt, sugar, saturated fats, chemicals, and additives. Reduce packaging waste and environmental pollution. Reduce killing of animals.

Objectives

Collect information about nutrition and health, new kitchen appliances, ingredients, and cooking processes. Understand and simplify the process of cooking. Create proper format for effective personal daily diet plan based on the information.

"I decided to call the personal daily diet plan DLC—1000+, which described clearly what I wanted to do. I wanted to eat a delicious, low-cholesterol diet with a calorie count of my choice, focused on my needs, convenience, concern for the environment, and taste.

"When I wrote it up and looked at it, I felt great." George announced with a proud smile.

"All of this seems too complicated to me. Did it work the way you wanted it to work? What did you find out later?" Farrah probed.

"Wait till we get there," replied George very quickly.

Desire and Empty Pocket

(Lack of Self-Confidence, Poor Self-Image)

Cassius: The fault, dear Brutus, is not in our stars,
but in ourselves, that we are underlings.

—WILLIAM SHAKESPEARE, IN *JULIUS CAESAR*

"This feeling of greatness was not to last long," George continued in a subdued voice. "As you probably know already, knowing something is one thing, and doing something about it is quite another.

"When my doubts cleared about what I wanted to do and what I should do, I was not cool, calm, confident, and self-assured like Arjun the great archer. Like him, I had realized what was important for me to do, however unpleasant it might be. But that is where the similarities stopped. There were quite a few obvious differences.

"Arjun had the most sophisticated weapons at his command. I did not even have a simple microwave oven.

"Arjun knew the enemies thoroughly. He knew who they were, what they could do, what their strengths and weaknesses were, and where and how they were likely to hide. He knew how to attack, when to attack, which weapons to use, how to use them, and why. He also knew the bad side effects of his powerful weapons.

"I did not know the basic ingredients for cooking or even the basics of the cooking process. I did not know about the latest medical thoughts and controversies in the ever-changing world of medical science.

"Arjun knew the technique; he had mastered the skills. He had spent the previous thirteen years learning more, acquiring more weapons, practicing, and polishing his skills. He had learned not only to endure the hardships but to overcome them.

"I had spent the past thirteen years enjoying and pampering my body and had forgotten what I had learned as a child.

"But now I was as determined as Arjun was; and now, like him, I also knew what I wanted to do.

"Based on the mission statement I had cooked up, the direction of my action was simple and straightforward. First, I posted the mission statement on my kitchen wall and also on the refrigerator. I decided to consult everyone possible to collect information regarding nutrition, ingredients, cooking processes, and menu building and to put all of that information into practice.

"*This should be simple and straightforward. You should be very proud of yourself. This should not take much time at all!* I assured myself.

"Gathering the medical information required a lot of time; it was pouring in continuously from so many sources. Collecting information on ingredients was tedious and time-consuming but interesting. Consulting friends and family to learn about the techniques of cooking, equipment, and so on was embarrassing and challenging, to say the least."

"Oh boy, that is a lot of challenge and a lot of hard work for sure. How did you find the time and energy to do all this?" bellowed James excitedly

"There is a very simple answer to that—my newfound enthusiasm, expectation of the reward of good health, and fear of consequences. I felt that all of this might not be simple, but it was exciting and rewarding. So I proceeded to work as hard as I could to collect all the necessary information, tools, and skills," George announced with a great deal of self-righteousness.

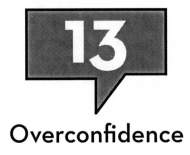

Overconfidence

*Pain nourishes courage; you cannot be brave if you
have had only wonderful things happen to you.*
—MARY TYLER MOORE

"How long did it take to do this, and did it work?" Ann asked. She had tried so many products and programs without long-term success and was always skeptical of any solutions.

"Ann, you are so smart," George whispered to Ann. He continued in his normal tone for the rest of the guests, "Here comes the interesting and important part of my education process! Now, I thought, I had investigated thoroughly, collected more than adequate data, and analyzed many different options. I felt that I had learned enough to do a good job of cooking and managing my diet and nutrition. I was absolutely confident about fixing a nice meal every day.

"Oh boy, was I wrong!

"We can laugh about it now, but that isn't how I felt on September

13 last year! Many of my friends had helped me collect information and learn about kitchen things, and I wanted to show what I had collected. It was my 'thank you' sort of event. In hindsight, you may say that I wanted to show off! Some of you may remember what happened. For those who were not here at that time, Joseph will fill you in with an unbiased description of my black September."

Joseph seemed only too eager to tell.

"George had called us at 6:00 p.m.," he said. "When Helen, Jason, Benjamin, Richard, and a couple of our other friends arrived at his house, only after several rings did George appear at the door. Mary, his wife, had called us earlier to let us know that she would be joining us later, so we weren't expecting her to be home. When George appeared at the door, he didn't exactly seem thrilled to see us come exactly on time; he said so in an awkward fashion, but we didn't catch the true meaning of it right then. He was quiet and somewhat nervous. As soon as he opened the door, my nose detected a strong, strange aroma in the air—pungent, aromatic, like something was burning, mixed in with a smell of some air freshener. I thought, *Wow, holy crap, what are we in for today?*

"After some uneasy exchanges of greetings, everyone looked at one another and became quiet. There was an awkward silence. In an attempt to get a lively conversation started, George tried to show us his recent collection of books, video programs, and different kitchen tools and equipment, including pots and pans of a special style. He then seated us at the table. It was very nicely decorated with new tableware, new hand towels, new placemats to match the tableware, and color-coordinated napkins. The conversation, however, was dull to say the least. The smell in the kitchen was so overpowering.

"The red wine was very good, and Richard complimented George on that, but that didn't do anything to his subdued mood. He tried to put on a brave face and began serving the items one by one. Then the trouble started.

"Jason had to miss his friend's birthday party to come with us, and he was already not too thrilled about being there. Jason was the only kid there. Helen and I had asked Jason to come with us because George was like an uncle to him, and we wanted Jason to see what George had accomplished. Jason was hungry and expecting a nice dinner; he couldn't stand the disappointment. He protested, 'I can't eat it. The rice is burned. Will you order me a pizza, Dad? I'm so hungry!' Helen tried to hush Jason, but it wasn't very effective.

"The food was all terrible. The vegetables were soggy, the salad had a little too much mint in it, the bean soup was watery and had too much salt, the other vegetable had too much garlic, and the flatbread had too much oil in it and was bitter and impossible to chew. All of us guests tried to keep up the polite front for a while, but it was no use.

"George accepted that the dinner was a bust. George also knew that ordering a pizza was a very simple solution to remedy the bad situation quickly. George ordered a large pizza with whatever toppings Jason wanted, to keep him happy, satisfied, and quiet. All of us enjoyed the pizza silently.

"After our pizza, Helen complimented George on his efforts and admired his collection of books and equipment. Richard and I gave him our friendly advice and encouraged him to try again. Jason thoroughly enjoyed the pizza and apologized to George for being so rude.

"Unfortunately, Jason couldn't keep himself quiet enough. 'Dad, tell Uncle George the story of the pundit and the boatman,' Jason insisted.

"It wasn't going to be a quiet evening. I tried to get out of telling the story, which was likely to be very offensive. 'It's too late, and we'd better be going home. George knows the story, and he has many other things to do,' I said to Jason sternly.

"George, however, was very happy that the dinner was over;

the diversion was God-sent and a perfect remedy for the disastrous evening. 'Please, Joe, tell us the story,' George insisted.

"Little did George know what he was getting into, and yet that story became the most important part of that evening for all of us dinner guests."

Robert raised his hand timidly. He wanted to ask a question but was not sure if he should interrupt the somber mood.

"What is it Robert?" asked Joseph.

"Some of us were not there and we missed that important story. We would love to hear it and learn from it. Will you share that story with us again?" enquired Robert.

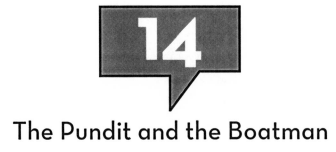

The Pundit and the Boatman

Appearances are deceitful.

—ANONYMOUS

Joseph took a sip of his coffee, cleared his throat, glanced at everyone present, and began telling the story again.

"Harold was a very learned man," he said. "He was born into a family of other learned men and women. Harold had spent a lot of time learning about history, geography, mathematics, philosophy, the arts, and the sciences known at that time. Harold knew a lot on every subject in the books. He had read a lot about India and the river Ganga in his books, and he was fascinated by what he had read. So one day Harold decided to visit India and experience the exotic beauty of those places he had read so much about.

"During one of his sight-seeing tours, Harold came to see the beauty and majesty of the river Ganga. He hired a boat to sail across the river. The small sailboat was operated by a poor, old sailor named Harry.

"Harry had never been to school.

"As Harold was chatting with Harry, it was obvious that Harry was weak at his grammar. Harold was shocked. He asked Harry if he had read Shakespeare.

"'No, my lord,' said Harry.

"'What! Not even one play?' asked Harold.

"'No, my lord, not a single one,' answered Harry.

"'But you have at least heard about the great Shakespeare, haven't you, my dear man?' asked Harold.

"'No, my lord, I have not heard about this great man of whom you speak so highly,' came the reply.

"Harold was very disappointed.

"'How about George Washington?' Harold asked.

"'No.'

"'Thomas Edison?'

"'No.'

"Then Harold asked Harry about history, geography, poetry, mathematics, and so on.

"Harry answered no to every question. Harry was honest and humble about it. Harold was greatly disappointed, but he tried not to let it show. He didn't want to hurt poor Harry's feelings.

"By this time, the boat had reached the middle portion of the mighty river. The gentle breeze suddenly changed into a strong gale. The clouds were getting darker, and a drop or two of rain fell. There was thunder and lightning in the sky above.

"Skinny, poor, old Harry looked at Harold and asked in his poor, broken English, 'Big storm coming, you know swim?'

"'No, my dear man, that is not the way you say it, and, yes, I know the various styles of swimming. I also know who won the gold medals in the last Olympics. I can tell you about the caloric expenditure in each event and the diets the athletes need.'

"By then Harold noticed that the boat was shaking and swerving,

45

and the boatman was having great difficulty controlling it. Harry looked up toward the sky and shouted again, 'You swim?'

"'May God help you with your English in your next life, my dear man, and if you mean, can I swim, the answer is *no*. I cannot.'

"'Then may God help you now, in this life,' said Harry as he jumped off the boat as it toppled over. With great difficulty and skill, Harry brought Harold to shore and saved his life. Harold was speechless for the next several months."

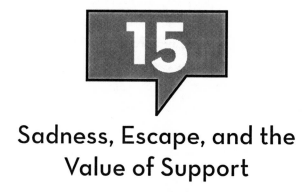

Sadness, Escape, and the Value of Support

Correction does much, but encouragement does more.
—JOHANN WOLFGANG VON GOETHE

"When I first finished telling that story," Joseph said, "everyone was quiet, wondering how George would take this direct but unintentional assault.

"George said, 'Thanks a million. I needed that. I realize now that it was fine to have an enlightened mind, books, and special pots and pans. That was the easy part.' And then he tried to put on a brave face."

"Looking back," George said, "even though I tried to put on a brave face, I was devastated. I felt miserable. I felt ashamed of my overconfidence, arrogance, and failure in front of my friends and colleagues. I was ready to give up. I never wanted to cook again. I didn't even want to try again. I felt that I just couldn't do it. I thought that I was not made for it. Everyone noticed my severe disappointment and setback.

"Edward tried to cheer me up. He said, 'George, there are many fine restaurants and cafeterias nearby where you could easily entertain your friends very well, without any hassle, apprehension, and uncertainty. Leave this cooking business to somebody else who has more time; you have more important things to do.'

"That didn't help at all. I was thinking, *How can I face my friends and colleagues at work tomorrow? How can I imagine inviting them for dinner at my home again in the future?* I was numb. I was standing near the door like a statue, except that I wasn't looking straight. I was looking down at the doorknob and the floor, wishing for everyone to leave and leave me alone.

"John had anticipated just such a scenario. John had seen many of his friends go through similar situations in the past. He had a rich collection of their stories. John said to me in a comforting voice, 'Not to worry, George. Cool it; calm down. You've come a long way; you're on the right track. Keep it up. Mishaps like this are just part of the process. Don't be discouraged; on the contrary, you should be proud of yourself. You recognized that your cooking skills need improvement. If what you're trying to do is important to you and something that you really want to do, you must be willing to face up to your challenge.'

"Richard was also encouraging; he said, 'George, John and I have met some people who will make you feel very comfortable because they have felt the way you're feeling today. They have gone through experiences like this. They continued their efforts and succeeded eventually. John and I have known some others who will make you feel proud of yourself for what you're doing because they gave up after just a single failed attempt; some others have given up after a few more failed attempts and have gone back to their old, wrong, unhealthy ways.

"'Some others, who were as discouraged in the past as you are now, will be eager to learn from you. Some are sitting on the fence and may give up if they see you give up. They may stay on and fight if you fight and show them the way. Some people here would love to share their experiences and what they went through before they succeeded.'

"When Richard stopped, I looked up, looked around, and realized that John and Richard were telling the truth. The sight of faces around me was positive proof. So I turned to John and asked, 'Please, John, whom have you met? Tell me their stories; tell me what problems they encountered and why I should feel proud when in reality I feel so bad.'"

Your Many Faces

We cannot become what we need to be
by remaining what we are.

—MAX DE PREE

John answered, "George, you've asked me many interesting questions in the past, but these new ones are very important. You ask, 'Why should I feel proud when in reality I feel so bad?'

"George, you should be proud of yourself because you have chosen a new path that will keep you healthy, and because you're not just talking about it; you're actually making an honest effort to put in practice what you've learned. What you're doing is not easy at all. It's definitely worthy of recognition and praise. And, I want to add that I'm proud of you, especially because you're curious and eager to learn from the experiences of others, instead of judging them one way or the other.

"You also ask, 'Whom have you met? Tell me their stories and what problems they encountered.'

"Do you remember chubby Charles?

"He does not know and does not want to know. An ignorant, blind, know-it-all, rich big shot, he is well travelled, prejudiced, and always looking down on the poor, skinny, malnourished people whom he has encountered during his travels. This is what he said to me the other day: 'Obesity indicates a good life and a good lifestyle. Obesity is not a problem, so there is no need to change.' When you run into him, he's likely to say to you, 'George, you don't know what you're talking about.' Charles is totally unable to see that the obese rich person is just as bad off as the starving poor.

"Do you know young, bubbly Bob?

"He does not know and does not want to know. He is ignorant, naive, young, and oblivious to the problems of obesity. He enjoys fat-people jokes, TV shows, and movies. You'll see him laughing at a TV movie about a fat person who is unable to balance his boxes of take-out food, while Bob is himself eating a pizza, a salad with a heap of creamy salad dressing, and ice cream or drinking beer. Bob is totally oblivious to the fact that his food and drink choices, if continued, will soon make him fat and miserable. Just ask him what he had for breakfast or lunch. Most likely, everything was rich in calories, with high fat, high salt, and very little fiber. And he'll insist that he ate a small amount of food!

"Do you know Jill?

"She does not know and is not sure if she wants to know. She wants to do something about her appearance. She is making little changes in her diet to look slim. She's doing something for a good reason, but she's doing it the wrong way. She's trying to eat small portions of high-calorie foods but avoids high-fiber foods and stays hungry and dissatisfied all the time. She's already looking at the possibility of liposuction, if what she's doing doesn't work. She has no faith in what she's doing. She's using the wrong method, which is full of problems, side effects, suffering, and complications, such as constipation, abdominal gas, bloating, pain, irregular habits, and poor sleep. Does she really want to know? Or is it only a superficial desire? Her goal seems to be only her looks and not health.

"Do you know Janet?

"She does not know and does not want to know. She wants to do something about her diet because everybody else is doing it, so she buys a lot of stuff based on the advertisements. Has it helped? No. What is her goal? She's bent on trying multiple products and multiple programs. She doesn't seem to have an interest in core principles. What she's doing is expensive and wasteful, and it's causing her a lot of frustration, anger, failure, and stress.

"Do you know Joyce?

"She does not know and isn't sure if she wants to know. She says, 'It looks nice that I'm making an effort. If it's not working, it's *not* my fault; I'm trying my best.' No dedication, no discipline, no real efforts to know.

"Do you know Joan?

"She says that she just wants to know. She has a bigger collection of diet books than yours. If you ask her why, she'll say, 'I'll use it *later!*'

"Do you know Jennifer?

"Jennifer just wants to know so she can talk about it, she admits.

"Do you know Tom?

"He knows a lot, and yet he cannot say no to chocolates, chips, cookies, and sugary drinks.

"Do you know Josephine?

"She wanted to know; she tried her best but gave up when she couldn't follow up with what was required. She had so many reasons for giving up.

"Do you know Jeremiah?

"He wants to know; he is trying his best and watching how you handle the situation.

"And I'm sure you've heard from others who have their own special reasons for not trying or for giving up after a short time. You,

George, are different. You want to know, to clarify your doubts, to remove your ignorance and confusion, to learn the skills, to take action, and to keep track of progress.

"Slipups are part of the process, so keep going," John said with genuine pride on his face.

Everyone was listening to John attentively, but it was getting very late. George was beginning to feel a little better. Now George had a real smile on his face and a suggestion. George said, "Why don't we break up for today and meet here again next Saturday? I'll try to do better next time. Are there any volunteers for cooking or for the stories?"

Even before George had finished his sentence, to everyone's surprise Jacob rushed forward. He was slim, tall, and handsome. Remember Jacob? After his college days, he put on a lot of weight and became really overweight. But look at him today. Earlier in the evening he had been standing in the back of the room, and yet he slipped quickly through between Josephine and Jeremiah.

"I'll be glad to help. I'll also tell the next story. I want everyone to listen to my story," Jacob said.

It seemed as if, by this time, everyone in the room wanted to share something important. It was written all over their faces.

Sueann wanted to tell about all her setbacks.

Linda wanted to tell who made her story possible.

Elizabeth wanted to tell about what had helped her the most.

That was great encouragement to George and many others. Even shy, sensitive, easily offended, easily discouraged, high-strung Ms. Dolittle wanted to share her story.

It was obvious that to let just Jacob or Ms. Dolittle take that volunteer spot would disappoint many others. That started a lot of whispering and brainstorming in the crowd. As always, John had a solution. He flipped a coin for a contest between Jacob and Ms. Dolittle. Ms. Dolittle won the toss.

Thus it was decided: first Ms. Dolittle, then Jacob, then everyone else.

Ms. Dolittle

The future belongs to those who believe
in the beauty of their dreams.
—ELEANOR ROOSEVELT

I grew up in a little town in rural Illinois. I was always slim, trim, smart, and pretty. My parents were strict. I was expected to help with many household chores. I used to help my mom wash dishes and do other chores, but cooking wasn't my favorite choice. Photography was my hobby, and that was my reward for doing the necessary chores. I was good in my studies in college, and I worked hard. I was ambitious. Finance and marketing were my favorite areas of study. After I finished college, I started to work for a financial firm in Chicago, a really busy place. Everyone was busy, busy, busy and businesslike—ambitious, aggressive, arrogant, and stressed. I had no time for anything except work. Even the fun was connected to work.

We ate out a lot. Breakfast was a quick donut—a different variety every day—or ham-and-egg-and-cheese biscuits, coffee, OJ, and so on. Lunch was hamburgers, pizza, quesadillas, special sandwiches, and a variety of salads with creamy dressings, and lots of soft drinks and coffee. Dinner was almost always a business affair in a restaurant with clients, with lots of wine and other tasty drinks and desserts. It was a very exciting life, indeed.

I lived in a fancy high-rise apartment overlooking Lake Michigan. "There's no chance of finding a real teacher here for me to learn how to cook," I assumed. Ready-to-eat food in a box, can, bottle, packet, or bag was always available within walking distance. Heat and eat, shake and bake, quick snacks, energy bars, energy drinks—whatever!

Over time, what do you think was the side effect of this "good life" of tasty, rich foods, plus wine and other beverages, plus desserts, plus mints, chocolates, and snacks in between?

My apartment complex had a gym and a swimming pool, but who had the time or desire to use them? Did I have the discipline to use them? Not me. I was ambitious. I was in a hurry to be the big shot. Without realizing it, I was becoming "big" for sure.

Occasionally I dreamed about cooking for myself, but when I chomped down on pizza on the weekends or a McMuffin on a Sunday morning, I immediately found so many reasons why I couldn't. The usual ones—no time, no information, no skills, and no help. The cookbooks that my mom and friends had given me were so complicated. The processes were so time-consuming. The ingredients were so numerous, and the quantity required was so difficult to measure unless I had all the measuring gadgets. Anyway, who was going to go to the store to find these special ingredients with a list in one's hand? It was so simple to just order from local restaurants—whatever I wanted, usually something that looked or sounded delicious online. I never paid attention to the complicated nutrition labels. One day someone made a comment about the labels: "The information is there for *you*, isn't it?" My response was, "Yes, if you're old or sick, or if your doctor tells you to read it." I thought I didn't have to look at the labels because I didn't need that information. Never was I interested in finding out why that information was placed there, why it was important, how I could use it, and why it would help me.

I wasn't aware of any change in my body, but one day, instead of being called "the skinny one," someone poked a finger at me and told me I was looking "prosperous." And I was stupid enough then to take it as a compliment! In reality, I later realized that I was rapidly on my way to becoming a model for one of Rubens's paintings. I looked around and noticed that everyone else at work was quite chubby, as well. That removed any discomfort I had felt about the "prosperous" comment and made me feel comfortable and okay with my new identity. Nobody at work talked about weight and diet too much, except to make fun of different weight-loss programs and the people who failed in their attempts to lose weight.

Everything would have gone on as usual, except one day I saw myself in one of the photographs a friend sent me. One of our coworkers was leaving to go to California, and someone had taken a lot of pictures at her going-away party. I was in some of those pictures. She had also included some of her pictures from California with her new coworkers. These pictures struck me like a thorn in both eyes at the same time! I wasn't used to looking at my photographs. I was the photographer and thus usually missed being in the picture myself.

What I saw in those pictures devastated me. I was upset; I was in turmoil. I couldn't imagine myself not being like those California girls. I struggled with myself for a solution. I didn't know what to do or how to handle it. I blamed my mom for not teaching me! I blamed it on my job and work environment. Once upon a time I had been worried about losing my job; now I wanted to get rid of my job and the work environment. I was ready to do whatever I could to change how I looked.

I wanted to be like the California girls in those pictures once more—bright, slim and trim, healthy and fit, vibrant and vivacious.

That was my inspiration.

I had to take the first step myself. I did.

All I had to do was *ask* for help. I did.

I started going to the gym. I found out that sixty-year-old Josh was more fit on the treadmill than I was. I also found out that he knew a lot about health, diet, fitness, and cooking. I didn't have specific information. He did. I didn't know why, when, or how. He did. I found out that good food probably costs less than restaurant food or processed, ready-to-eat energy bars and snacks. My mom was excited to know that I wanted to learn. I found out how enjoyable it can be.

I didn't have to give up my job or blame anyone or anything. I learned to deal with it. I learned to respect myself and my values. When my colleagues saw the "changing me," I was an inspiration to at least two of my colleagues. Can you imagine how proud that makes me feel?

So, George, your success is in your hands. Keep it up. You're on the right path, and when you're on the right path you'll sooner or later get to your destination. Don't be discouraged. When you don't know the way, do not be afraid to ask for help.

Jacob

Nobody can stop the man with the right mental attitude from achieving his goal, and nothing on Earth can help the man with the wrong mental attitude.

—THOMAS JEFFERSON

Everyone's eyes were now focused on Jacob.

All of us dinner guests had known Jacob since his childhood. He had been a good student but wasn't exactly focused on studying to get the best grades. He was more interested in sports and music, fancy clothes, fun things, and living a "good life." He was quite handsome, athletic, and always curious. He seemed like a happy-go-lucky guy, always the life of a party. He could sure put down some beers! He seemed confident, bold, and sometimes even outright arrogant and boastful—always independent, doing things his own way. He was the know-it-all, smart-aleck type but was almost always bubbly and friendly. He had the "I know everything, everybody else sucks, I don't care, it doesn't matter" attitude.

As the years passed, we noticed some changes. Jacob put on quite a bit of weight; he became quieter, slower in his movements, more aloof, and less bubbly—almost a loner. Now, however, he looked better than ever—humble, polite, quiet, and happy in a different way. George was very interested in his story.

"I did it *my* way. All of you have known me for a long time, but not really," Jacob said boldly.

"As you all know, I was good in math, marketing, and computer skills, so I decided to be an IT professional. Because I was assertive and lucky, I found a great job. There was no limit to 'bigger and better' and the stress that results from it. I was bubbly on the outside and sad inside. I had no balance and no peace. I had a different way of looking at things. I felt that I had a right to do as I pleased. I felt that I had a right to enjoy anything possible to get happiness and peace, which I felt I deserved.

"You may now call that a misplaced freedom and misplaced sense of thrill and happiness. I felt that nothing else tasted better than a different ice cream after each meal or a juicy Omaha steak with a full bottle of the finest red wine every Tuesday. And I better not talk about the weekends!

"Who cared what might happen later? Life was for living. Who knew what tomorrow would bring? Tomorrow would take care of itself; I wanted to be bold, live on the edge, and get the thrill while I could. This is what I always told myself. These pseudo-scientific explanations drowned out simple, sane, polite opposition from friends and family.

"I could see that I was putting on weight. I had to buy new clothes quite frequently; my shirt-collar size was changing month by month, and also my belt size. I would have liked to be slimmer just to fit into my expensive clothes! I couldn't run. I was gasping for breath when I tried to walk quickly or use stairs. But I did not or would not pay attention to these simple facts.

"I was trying in the beginning, whenever I saw a new advertisement about a new program, and I failed many times. Failing bothered me at first. After some time, however, failures stopped bothering me. It was obvious. It was "their" fault. Their product was no good. So I tried another product and yet another. No success. No peace. Then a feeling came over me: 'Hey, I'm doing my best. It's not working, but there's not much more that I can do. So be it.' I told myself that I was made to be overweight and that there was nothing wrong with it. It was just my bad luck. I continued on the wrong track.

"No patience, no guidance, no consistency, no faith, no supportive feedback. Stop, go, change, good results, no results, bad results, frustration, anger, hopelessness, and continuous turmoil. So I just let it happen and stopped thinking much about it. I pushed it out of my mind any way I could. 'Go away and leave me alone,' I said often to my thought-making machine (myself).

"Immediate pleasure to seek happiness was my standard reaction, with the same poor results. I thought that a good cheesecake, a great steak, and a bottle of wine or beer was the way to comfort my stressed mind, something to fill up the 'hole in the soul.'

"I was thirsty for something and running after the mirage. I couldn't listen to the wise, old companion telling me that the mirage has no ability to quench my thirst. I was hurting, but my pride prevented me from expressing the truth, seeking proper advice, or asking questions. I had a great fear of consequences and also a fear of failure.

"All of this is my evaluation in retrospect. I didn't see my behavior in this way at that time. I was trying 'my way.' I was so 'smart' (or arrogant). I was confident that I would fix it soon, that it wasn't necessary to ask for help.

"People called me inflexible, stubborn, obstinate, unyielding, stupid, and ignorant. I looked at it differently. I was hiding and avoiding 'them.' I concluded that I was made to be this way. I was ignoring all the warning signs. I was afraid of failure and yet kept on sandbagging myself with ice cream to keep me happy, with granola bars to give me energy, or with a beer or two to give me courage! I was cheating myself and my well-wishers.

"To avoid loneliness, I spent a lot of time on the Internet. One day, I met this girl online. Besides IT stuff, our chat extended to travel, movies, music, and sports. She rode mountain bikes. That led sometimes to talk about restaurants, food, fitness, and health. I was impressed by her knowledge, charm, gentleness, and discipline. She was vibrant and enthusiastic. We enjoyed discussing the challenges of new technology at work and each other's scientific skills. She made me feel great and at ease. She became my best friend. She e-mailed me her photographs. I avoided sending my photograph. I gave excuses, delayed, and finally flatly refused. I was afraid to meet her in person because of my weight. At the same time, I couldn't imagine losing her for any reason, especially my stupidity, arrogance, or weight problem. I was determined to have her as my life partner.

"That was my inspiration and my challenge to change. I was slowly waking up to the fact that by trying on my own, I was sandbagging myself. I was worried to death. Because I was now committed to my goal, I asked myself: How can I get in shape? How can I give up the things I grew up with? How can I ask someone to help me? Me? Ask someone for something? Can I be that humble? Can I be accountable to someone else? What about everyone laughing at me when I stumble? Who is there to support me and encourage me if I falter or fail?

"Finally I recognized that even if I didn't want to learn to cook like a gourmet chef, I could certainly learn from someone that I trusted and respected and could be accountable to."

"Who can that be? Your girlfriend?" Benjamin jumped in with impatience and excitement.

"No. Not my girlfriend. My grandmother," shot back Jacob. "I decided that I could certainly learn from my grandmother and my computer, to build my own diet plan with the items available in local stores. When I asked my grandmother, she was shocked but very happy to show me her way. She was old-fashioned, hardworking, disciplined, and tough as nails—wiry, slim, and straight. She gave me what I needed the most—encouragement, reassurance, and advice to be patient. She helped me stay on the right path. I began to eat more oatmeal and fewer biscuits and gravy, more raw or steamed broccoli and less mashed potatoes with extra butter, more grapes and less wine. It wasn't easy. It was neither pleasant nor quick, but now I was accountable to my grandmother, whom I respected, trusted, and loved. She was tough on me but didn't belittle me and was always encouraging. All of you can see that being accountable to my grandmother has worked very well for me.

"George, if I can help in any way, please feel free to let me know. Our God-given gift of life—or GGG—is too important for us to just let it slip out of our hands because of the excuses we give ourselves. GGG is our responsibility to protect," Jacob concluded, to thunderous applause and tears of joy.

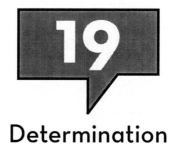

Determination

The basic difference between an ordinary man and a warrior
is that a warrior takes everything as a challenge, while an
ordinary man takes everything either as a blessing or a curse.

—DON JUAN

George was beginning to feel better.

"Great fight. Great story. Great help. Your story will bring me back on track, no matter what demons and obstacles I face," said George with renewed determination.

It was past midnight when Jacob stopped telling his story. Everyone had been listening to the tale of his struggles, obstacles, despair, courage, and triumph and the outpouring of his deepest thoughts and feelings. Nobody had thought that it had been this difficult. Everyone was shocked by Jacob's story and frightened by Jacob's struggle. After the initial applause, there was a period of dead silence. Everyone was numb.

After a short period, they began to reflect on their recent past. Richard opened up. Richard lived in a metropolitan area and had always blamed his weight problem on that. He said, "I was surprised at the ups and downs Jacob had to go through. I know what it is to feel up one day and down the next, and what that does to my eating habits."

Edward admired Jacob for his computer skills. Edward was always meticulous with his work. He also liked his ritual of eating at Mexican restaurants every Saturday and Italian, Chinese, and steakhouse restaurants in between. Edward said, "I never thought Jacob would stick with and win his fight with *his* eating and drinking habits!"

James apologized. He said to Jacob, "I feel so bad now for laughing at you when you were clumsy, huffing and puffing and trying to dance."

Helen said, "I'm ashamed of myself for criticizing you when you had setbacks.

John said, "I feel so stupid now for making sly remarks about your habit of buying new clothes every few months when you were actually struggling with a problem."

Debra said, "I couldn't stand your arrogance when you told me the information about calories, fats, and complex carbs; I felt that you were just full of—you know what, all talk and no action."

Jacob smiled and accepted their apologies gracefully. Jacob had shown them that it could be done. Each one hugged Jacob, thanked him, and said, "We're all grateful to you for showing us that it can be done. We feel inspired by the fighting spirit, hard work, and perseverance you showed." Jacob smiled, appreciating the new response from his friends and said, "I have just one more important point I want to tell you. When you fumble in your goal, don't ever condemn yourself. Correct the mistake and move on."

But even as they heard Jacob say that, George's guests were heavy with thoughts of their own struggles, and they had the same lingering questions on their mind. Richard wondered, "Jacob did it, but can I do it with the burden of all *my* problems?" Edward thought, "Do I *really* need to change my eating habits?" Helen felt, "Do I really need to *go through* this pain and suffering?"

Benjamin wanted to congratulate Jacob on his success, call him a lucky guy, and leave it at that, with a hidden feeling of "Why can't I be so lucky?"

It seemed as if nobody wanted to leave just yet, but everyone had to get ready for work in a few hours. The guests had a lot of heated and spirited discussions, arguments, comments, and opinions, and in the end everyone was pumped up and charged to fight his or her battle.

Richard said, "Improving eating habits is important."

Edward announced, "Each one has to find his or her own way."

Benjamin declared, "Each one has to find and fight his or her demons and obstacles."

Everyone agreed that it is *not* easy, but it *can* be done.

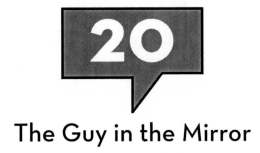

The Guy in the Mirror

Friend: One who knows all about you and loves you just the same.
—ELBERT HUBBARD

"**D**essert for anyone?" inquired George in a loud, booming, clear voice, bringing all of us dinner guests from the past to the present. George was beaming from ear to ear with the well-deserved smile of a winner.

"Of course. Roll it down. We're ready for dessert," echoed everyone present.

"I sure did learn a lot on that black September day," declared George as he was serving his special mixed-fruit dessert.

While George was busy doing that, someone pointed at the décor in George's kitchen. George had a vast collection of books, videos, CDs, and DVDs on shelves. He had cookbooks, diet books, medical textbooks, and travel magazines. He had specialized tools and gadgets and the latest kitchen appliances.

Catherine was overwhelmed. Chatting with Doris, she wondered, "Must I have all these things to start or to be successful? Do I have to read all these books? Do I have to get all this information? How necessary are all these things? Can I begin without so much start-up cost?"

John recognized the whispers. He knew the feelings of the nervous fence-sitters.

So he asked, "George, what do you really need to be successful? Was it the equipment, or was it something else? Was it the information or the skills? What was the most important factor?"

George didn't want to be bashful. He replied, "John, you know what I've gone through over the years. What have *you* observed me going through? Please tell our friends what you've noticed as an outsider."

John directed the question to Richard. "Richard, what did you notice?"

Richard said, "George acknowledged his lack of knowledge and accepted that. He got over his fear of asking questions. He struggled with his doubts and didn't give up on himself."

John then asked Edward, "What did you notice?"

Edward said, "George recognized that his health—his God-given gift—is the most precious. The recognition of this fact inspired George and motivated him to do everything to protect and preserve it. George took action. He worked hard, kept focus, faced obstacles, and persisted."

Joseph said, "George remained determined and kept his faith that God was on his side. Nobody else told him to do it. He continued on the journey that he himself had initiated. George continues to do what is required each and every day."

John summarized, "In short, information, desire, wishes, dreams, money, advisers, tools, and gadgets are all fine; that's the easy part. Ultimately, you have to work with what you already have and build from there. You have to act and get your hands dirty; you have to anticipate and be ready for the falls. You'll get angry and frustrated at yourself. You'll have to pull yourself back up, again and again. To eat healthfully is the most important responsibility you have toward yourself, to protect the GGG. The sooner you recognize and accept that, the better off you'll be. So, George, tell us now in your own words. Simplify it further for us: How were you able to do this?"

George said, "As everyone knows, all of us have a long list of instant answers for why it can't be done. Instead, we must ask ourselves what is necessary and how it *can* be done.

"Each one of us has to decide on the destination.

"Each one of us has to find the inspiration to do that.

"Each one of us has to continue to make honest efforts and always remember what Thomas Jefferson said a long time ago: 'The harder I work, the luckier I get.'"

George paused for a moment and then asked, "Richard, what do you think of the guy in the mirror? Do you love the guy in the mirror? Are you his best friend? Do you look out for his best interests? Can you be honest with him?

"Then, here is an important suggestion. You, Richard, must do what you would like the guy in the mirror to do! It's crucial that you understand, love, and respect the guy in the mirror. If you don't understand, love, and respect the guy in the mirror, you must find out why and figure out how you will change that.

"Telling the guy in the mirror to just say no is *not* enough! Your actions get the job done, and for that you must develop a positive mind-set about yourself."

The Roadmap

(If You Want to Go to New York ...)

Always bear in mind that your own resolution to
succeed is more important than any one thing.

—ABRAHAM LINCOLN

"**G**eorge, did you ever get angry at the guy in the mirror? Did you ever cheat on your diet and condemn yourself for it? Did you ever get sad and depressed when you gained a few pounds, instead of losing?" Ann asked cautiously.

"Friends, to tell you the truth, every time I had a setback, even a minor failure, I felt that it was a disaster," George admitted with great humility. "It made me feel bad, sometimes for a short time and sometimes for days. I used to get discouraged quite easily, but I wasn't ready to give up—on my efforts or on myself.

"Giving up sure seemed tempting as a quick impulse, but then I always asked, 'What will I gain in the long run?' The answer was crystal clear—nothing good on that road. Accepting this thought in my heart helped me block that road each time I had a temptation to do otherwise. Whenever I had the impulse to complain or blame someone or something else, I found out that the listeners were only other unhappy, discouraged people, and they weren't fun to be with for long. I wasn't going to be on that road.

"I'll never forget the lesson from my high-school geography teacher: 'If you want to go to New York, get a map and start on the road to New York, not on the road to Texas. If you stay on the road to New York, slowly but surely that road will take you where you want to go.'

"I had decided on my 'destination.' I wanted to eat right. So obviously I needed a roadmap. As you already know, I had collected all kinds of information. Now I was excited about the journey and dreaming of the great things that I was sure waited for me at the destination. I started learning about ingredients and about the process of cooking. It wasn't easy, but that is what I did. Whenever someone was willing to teach me something about cooking, I was willing and ready to learn."

"How did you do that?" Joann questioned.

George had a bold answer. He said, "Like an eager beaver, I observed others whenever the opportunity presented itself. I know many great cooks. Like a starving beggar asks for food, I asked for answers to my questions about cooking. Sometimes I received good answers, and sometimes I got ridiculed. Whenever someone was willing to teach me something about cooking, I was willing to learn.

"Every time I put a morsel in my mouth, wherever I was, I asked myself, 'What is it? What ingredients can I identify? What cooking processes must have gone into its making? Is it good for me? Do I need it? How much sugar? How much salt? How much fat? How much oil? How much cholesterol is there in this recipe?' You'll be surprised how easy it is to find out this information and how shocking it can be.

"I didn't want to impress somebody else with my cooking. I just wanted to use the medical information I had collected, along with information about cooking, to improve my own eating habits without disregarding taste and convenience. That's how I came to appreciate the complexities of cooking. That's how I also came to realize the simplicity of it all.

"Now I was ready to take the next step: develop my own parameters to put it all together to dictate my eating style. That is exactly what I did with John's help. John will explain the details to you."

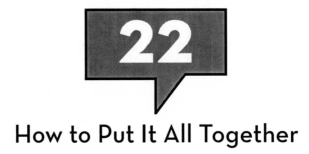

How to Put It All Together

*Nothing can withstand the power of the human will if it is
willing to stake its very existence to the extent of its purpose.*
—BENJAMIN DISRAELI

The following are George's parameters to dictate the eating style
for anyone who wants to protect the privilege of healthy life:

» The eating style must be nutritionally sound and based on
need.

» The eating style must include tasty choices.

» The eating style must be convenient.

» The eating style must have variety.

» The eating style must meet the Dietary Guidelines for
Americans, as developed by the Center for Nutrition Policy
and Promotion, an organization of the US Department of
Agriculture.

» The eating style must clearly track information on calories, fats, sugars, and salts.

» The eating style must create as little environmental damage as possible.

» The eating style must leave room for choice, indulgence, and impulse.

» The eating style must be satisfying.

George dubbed his eating style NEET:

» *nutrition*—cannot compromise because it is the basic principle

» *ease, simplicity, and convenience*

» *environment*—must always keep ourselves aware of the environmental impact of everything we do and protect the environment the best way we can

» *taste*—cannot compromise because we will not be successful in our task otherwise; however, the taste is mostly acquired, so we must create a balance in our eating style, with special regard to the taste

Helen, Justin, and a few others were getting a little restless, as if they had something very important on their minds but weren't quite sure how to bring it up. They were just looking at each other, and then Sueann took the initiative and spoke up.

"The big challenge is always *how* to implement these guidelines? I have a lot of questions that need to be answered before this can be done. Words are fine on a piece of paper, but how do you implement this in real life?" Sueann nervously handed a long list of her questions to George and requested he ask John to clarify some of these points.

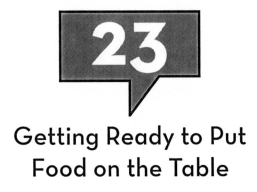

Getting Ready to Put Food on the Table

Do what you can, with what you have, where you are.

—THEODORE ROOSEVELT

John always welcomed questions. He never belittled George or anyone else for asking simple questions. So when George wanted to do things in a NEET way, he asked John many questions, and John answered them all. Here is how it went.

Why do we eat?

We need energy (fuel) to survive, build our body, and function every day. We eat to get the needed energy and the necessary building materials. We also eat to enjoy the taste as a form of entertainment and pleasurable activity.

How do we measure this energy (Fuel) in food?

Calories are the unit of measurement for this energy in food.

How much energy (calories) do we need every day?

That number is different for different individuals. You may want to ask your healthcare provider to advice you on the calorie number suitable for you.

Is there a difference in the energy we get from an apple, a glass of milk, or a hamburger?

The energy is the same, but the *amount of energy and building material* in an apple is different than in a glass of milk or a hamburger. The amount of energy depends on the amount of macronutrients, such as carbohydrates, fats, and proteins, in the food. One gram of carbohydrates has four calories, one gram of fat has nine calories, and one gram of protein has four calories.

How do we find out the amount of energy (calories) in any food item?

Read the nutrition label, search for the food online, or get a book or smartphone app with information about calorie count. Google the question: How many calories in xxx?

What should we eat?

We should eat whatever gives us that needed energy (Fuel), the building material and other necessary ingredients such as the fiber, vitamins etc.

How much should we eat?

We should eat enough to fulfill our need for energy (fuel, number of calories) and building materials *and also to create a sense of satisfaction or fullness.*

75

How do we prepare food and get it ready to put on the table to eat?

Some foods can be eaten raw or unprocessed. Some foods require processing before they can be eaten. Cooking is the process of preparing food for eating.

Why do we cook?

We cook food to make it taste better, to make it easier to digest, to make it look better and enhance the visual appeal, to incorporate ingredients together, and to make it safe.

Do we have names for these processes and for the resulting products?

Yes. We eat food that is unprocessed, as in methods one through six, or processed, as in methods seven through nineteen.

1. Fresh (e.g., as in fresh vegetables)
2. Unripe, raw (e.g., raw or green mango or green banana)
3. Ripe (e.g., ripe mango or yellow banana)
4. Frozen (e.g., frozen yogurt)
5. Dry (e.g., dried apricots, dates, figs, etc.)
6. Mix
7. Bake (to prepare food using dry heat, often in an oven)
8. Steam (to apply heat in the form of steam)
9. Simmer (to apply low-grade heat with food and water just under the boiling point)
10. Boil (to apply heat to food and water until the mixture boils)
11. Puree (to apply heat or mechanical means to soften food)
12. Roast (to apply dry heat to remove moisture)

13. Broil (to apply heat directly above or below a food)

14. Barbecue (to apply heat to food that is on a rack so the fat can dribble away)

15. Pan broil (to cook over direct heat in an uncovered skillet)

16. Fry (to heat food in different amounts of fat)

    Deep fry = +++ oil

    Shallow fry = ++ oil

    Stir fry/sauté = + oil

17. Marinate (to soak food in a liquid mixture to improve its flavor and/or texture)

18. Smoke (to roast and flavor food using smoke)

19. Glaze (to cover food with sauce, syrup, or another liquid coating)

Many of these processes sound complicated and time-consuming. Can we use simple processes for now?

If we understand the underlying process, we can do the cooking differently. Understanding the processes helps us choose *what we eat, how we process it, and how we use the simpler and less time-consuming processes.* Simple cooking processes involve adding heat, adding or removing water, adding or removing fat, and adding taste enhancer(s).

In most cooking, food is heated.

Sometimes water is removed a little.

Sometimes water is removed a lot or completely.

Sometimes water is added a little.

Sometimes water is added a lot.

Sometimes oil or fat are added.

Sometimes oil or fat are removed.

Sometimes while heating another ingredient is added by the source of heat, such as smoke from wood.

Sometimes several ingredients are mixed together.

Sometimes in addition to the basic heat, water, and oil, another taste enhancer is added.

Occasionally food is processed differently; instead of adding heat, food is cooled, chilled, or frozen.

Just to show it graphically, here is how it looks:

Ingredient	Process			Taste Enhancer
Main ingredient	**Add heat**	**Add water**	**Add oil or fat**	Add additional ingredient(s)
	Decrease temperature (freeze)	**Remove water**	**Remove oil or fat**	Add taste enhancer(s)

Are there any tools that we can use for processing our food to create this advantage (adding heat, adding or removing water, adding or removing fat, adding taste enhancers)?

All of this can be done using the microwave and new types of food processors.

What are taste enhancers?

They are additional agents added to the main ingredient to improve or change the taste and flavor of the recipe. People have used these agents for many, many years throughout the world.

Examples include salt, lemon juice, sugar, herbs and spices, soy sauce, commercial dips and spreads, jams/jellies/preserves, and many other products.

For example, to make a simple spinach dish using the microwave, you can follow these steps:

1. Unpack a pack of frozen spinach and place it in a bowl. Cover it with a microwave-safe lid.
2. Zap it for five minutes.
3. Remove from the microwave and add a taste enhancer.
4. Enjoy your ready-to-eat item.

The diagram shows the process in a pictorial way.

How to Make Simple Meal Items

Choose main ingredient (such as frozen spinach, broccoli, or potato)	Add heat (microwave using a lid)	Add water (choose the amount)	Add oil or fat (such as olive oil, butter, sour cream, etc.)	Add additional ingredients and taste enhancers (such as lemon juice and salt)

By changing the amount of time, heat, fat, or oil and adding a different taste enhancer, you can change the taste of your spinach dish as many times as you want and create many spinach items to satisfy your tongue. If you add the calories in the spinach and the flavor enhancer, you know the total calories in that item.

You can also choose a different vegetable instead of spinach and process it in a similar way to create multiple items with different tastes. Try it; you'll like it.

Create a different taste for broccoli, spinach, or any other vegetable each time you process it. Make it more interesting and tasty each time, just the way you want it. Make eating vegetables simple and tasty.

Another useful gadget is a food processor to puree fruits and vegetables together with milk or yogurt to create your own recipe.

The idea seems fascinating and useful, but you no doubt have many more questions. How do I choose the ingredients? Which process do I use for which ingredient? For how much time should I add heat? How do I add or remove the water, and how much? How and when do I add or remove the fat, and how much? Which fat should I add? Which taste enhancer? How much? When? How much time will it need? What if I don't like the taste? Will I have to throw it all away?

With time, patience, experiments, and practice, George gradually found his own answers, and so will you.

How do I choose the ingredients?

Choose three or four different vegetables daily. Prepare each vegetable with a different process, or use the same vegetable with different taste enhancers. Use leftovers with different processes or different taste enhancers. Just make sure that you don't use the same ingredients too often.

How do I choose the cooking process?

Use any simple process, from one to eleven.

How do I choose the taste enhancer?

Begin with the simplest ones (salt, pepper, sugar, lemon juice, or a prepared sauce) and grow. Experiment with small amounts. When in doubt, use simpler methods.

How do I know which process to use for which ingredient?

Use trial and error: go slow and consult the many recipe books available in the market.

What if I don't like the taste of the vegetable?

Begin with simple steaming and increase to complex mixtures and frying. Try a teaspoon of olive oil as a taste enhancer and modify as needed.

How much time will it take to prepare?

If you buy ready-to-use ingredients, such as canned beans and precut frozen vegetables, you can save a great deal of time, but watch out for the sodium content and environmental impact of the containers and packaging materials.

What else do beginners need to learn?

Different processes enhance the flavor, texture, and palatability of different ingredients differently. Some processes work better with some ingredients. And sometimes there's no better teacher than a little trial and error—for example, baking the beans to a crisp charcoal or boiling the rice to a soggy mush.

Use a simple, straightforward process in the beginning and, as you become proficient, increase the complexity according to your individual abilities and desires.

Taste is such a personal thing. Our tongues do universally enjoy fat, salt, and sugar, but taste is mostly an acquired phenomenon. One person dripping with sweat and slurping his delicious curry may turn off a Westerner, while a person chomping on her rare, juicy, pink steak may churn the stomach of an Easterner. When you're ready to cook, keep in mind the basic principle that taste is a personal thing, and you've won half the battle.

What gives us the satiety, the sense of fullness and satisfaction?

This is a very important question, and I do not have a very definite, scientific answer. I feel that each individual has to search within himself or herself to find out how he or she gets satiety. Then you have to learn how to use that knowledge to your advantage in designing your eating style and creating the balance.

Is exercise important along with calorie count in managing weight?

If you don't use it, you lose it! We need exercise to maintain and build muscle mass, build strength, keep flexibility, and remain fit for our day-to-day activities. When one is trying to lose weight, a combination of exercise and proper diet helps to create the necessary energy deficit to reduce weight.

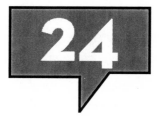

Building the Personal Daily Diet Plan

You get what you inspect, not what you expect.
—MANAGEMENT ADAGE

D ebra raised her hand. She had a question, and now she didn't feel embarrassed to ask about anything that was important to her. She asked, "I have read many recipe books and realized that one recipe does not make the total picture. So, George, what did you do beyond learning to make simple items? Do you have a plan to create a total picture for every day and from day to day?"

"Right on, Debra. Glad you asked that. I was wondering about the same thing," chimed in Helen.

George had already done just that.

After George learned how to prepare an individual item for eating and what the cooking process involved, he wanted to develop a program for himself and others to eat several times a day, from day to day and in different environments.

When he recognized that his intake should be based on need, ease, environment, and taste (NEET) to keep himself and the environment healthy, everything else followed automatically.

Your goal: eat better every day. In other words, eat NEET.

To do that, you must first find out your individual caloric and nutritional needs. You already have general guidelines to help you with that. You know that to gain weight you must take in excess calories, and to lose weight you must take in fewer calories than your body uses. To maintain weight, you must keep a balance. Calories taken in must equal calories used. We're talking about weight over a period of time and the total caloric intake during that period. And remember that we are talking about the *energy* (fuel) intake from the food as well as the building materials, and not the *amount* of food.

MyPlate, a program developed by the Center for Nutrition Policy and Promotion, a program of the US Department of Agriculture, gives general guidelines about important nutrition factors. To build your personal daily diet plan, you must keep it simple. Many people divide the daily intake of food into several categories, such as breakfast, lunch, dinner, and snacks, which is fine. You may like to eat a big breakfast and a big lunch, and your spouse may like to eat a small breakfast and a big lunch. Each individual's habits and needs are different. What you really need to do is carefully pay attention to the total amount of calories taken in during the day and from day to day. You must monitor both the calories and the distribution of the sources of these calories: the fats, proteins, complex carbohydrates, refined carbohydrates, and simple sugars, as well as the salt, fiber, and other important factors in the food.

Sounds tedious, doesn't it? It's not that difficult when you learn the tricks.

Everyone has a personal daily diet plan. Sometimes it's thrust upon you by your schedule. Sometimes it's controlled by your work environment. Sometimes it's recommended by your health-care provider. Most of the time, though, it's decided by your nose, your tongue, and your available time, unfortunately with total disregard for calories and the distribution of those calories.

Without a written diary of food intake or an excellent memory, it's not easy to keep track of what you're doing and not doing. If you're like most people, you assemble foods from different recipes at different times and in different amounts. You eat without trying to remember accurately what you ate earlier that day.

Here is the Golden Rule: Create your own daily diet plan and a process to keep track of your daily food intake, at least until you feel comfortably efficient and effective without one. Use the diet planner to create a simple structure for your personal daily diet plan. It allows you to automatically monitor the sources and distribution of calories, other nutritional requirements, and total energy (calorie) intake. Don't forget that having variety in your diet is important to ensure that all your nutritional needs are well taken care of. Many experts have recommended many different distributions of macronutrients for daily energy (calorie) intake. This table shows how those recommendations vary:

Carbohydrates	45 percent to 65 percent
Proteins	10 percent to 35 percent
Fats	20 percent to 35 percent

The critical issue isn't the relative proportion of macronutrients in the diet, so long as there are no extremes. What's important is to ensure that you get an adequate intake of all the necessary nutrients, keeping in mind taste and satiety. You decide what you want to eat and when and where you want to eat it; understand what each food contains and be aware of the sources and calories.

You decide the source of your fats. You decide the source of your proteins. For these macronutrients (fats and proteins), please learn about the advantages and disadvantages of getting them from either plant or animal sources. Reduce simple sugars and refined carbohydrates in your diet. You decide what is satisfying for you. If you monitor the total number of calories (energy) taken in and maintain it according to your need, your plan will work. Diets with a wide range of macronutrient proportions have been documented to promote weight loss and prevent weight regain after loss.

Create a total picture for every day by choosing items from A and B.

A) Meal items you prepare yourself

B) Meal items you obtain from elsewhere: the supermarket shelf, a restaurant, a neighbor, leftovers, and so on

Use the personal daily diet planner. Fill in the boxes and count the approximate calories for each box, keeping in mind the importance of variety in the diet. Use a special app on your smartphone, Google, or any other calorie-counting gadget to get the approximate count on the calories in the items you choose.

Personal Daily Diet Planner				
For breakfast, lunch, dinner, and snacks			Date: [Yesterday]	
	Process	Ingredient	Amount	Calories
Juice/soft drink				
Milk/dairy				
Fruits				
Cereal				
Vegetable	Fresh			
Vegetable	Steamed			
Vegetable	Boiled			
Vegetable	Baked			
Vegetable	Fried			
Vegetable	Marinated			
Vegetable	Dried			
Vegetable	Mixed			
Beans				
Tree nuts and seeds				
Bread				
Rice/pasta				
Oil/butter/fats				
Condiments/ snacks/ chips/ chocolate/etc.				
Dessert				
Alcohol				
Meat/poultry/fish				
Extra (your favorite item)				
		Total Calories ------>		

Personal Daily Diet Planner				
For breakfast, lunch, dinner, and snacks			Date: [Today]	
	Process	Ingredient	Amount	Calories
Juice/soft drink				
Milk/dairy				
Fruits				
Cereal				
Vegetable	Fresh			
Vegetable	Steamed			
Vegetable	Boiled			
Vegetable	Baked			
Vegetable	Fried			
Vegetable	Marinated			
Vegetable	Dried			
Vegetable	Mixed			
Beans				
Tree nuts and seeds				
Bread				
Rice/pasta				
Oil/butter/fats				
Condiments/ snacks/ chips/ chocolate/etc.				
Dessert				
Alcohol				
Meat/poultry/fish				
Extra (your favorite item)				
		Total Calories ------>		

Step-by-step guide

1. Each individual must fill out one for himself or herself, each day.

2. Begin with filling out the form based on the food intake *yesterday*.

3. Do this for several days; create a habit.

4. Count the total calories approximately.

5. Decide on the approximate number of calories you want to eat today.

6. Make sure you have adequate variety in your selections.

7. Choose the amount for each item.

8. Fill out the approximate number of calories for each item.

9. Calculate the total calories for the day.

10. The column marked "favorite" is only for emergencies or indulgences, so keep it empty as much as possible.

11. The amount and quality of the fat, butter, or oil should be clearly identifiable.

When you eat a variety of ingredients and use a variety of processes, the nutritional adequacy of your diet is mostly assured.

With a predominantly vegetarian diet and with dairy products, a high-fiber, low-fat, protein-adequate, low-cholesterol, low-salt, high-calcium diet is mostly assured. If you feel an irresistible need for animal protein, add it with the knowledge of the additional caloric, nitrogen, fat, and cholesterol burden. Lean toward cooked, dry beans and nuts instead of meat and fish for adequate protein intake.

Create a new taste that you enjoy, every day.

By making the building blocks clearly identifiable, you know where and what to eat, how much to cut, what to avoid, and how much to indulge.

Don't worry about being perfect; keep on the road, and it will take you where you want to go.

Using the personal daily diet plan provides the following benefits:

» It forces you to think and plan for the whole day and from day to day.

» It makes you aware that you need variety in your diet.

» It helps you monitor your daily caloric intake.

» It lets you decide on the variety of tastes you wish to include: hot, medium, mild, or bland.

» It helps you monitor your salt intake and its sources.

» It helps you monitor your fat intake and its sources.

» It helps you monitor your sugar intake and its sources.

» It helps you monitor your protein intake and its sources.

» It guides you to be on the right track.

» It keeps you in control.

Remember, this isn't a cookbook for exotic, complex recipes, but you can add whatever you want to the personal daily diet plan, so long as you keep whatever you desire within your nutritional needs and energy requirements. The NEET method (nutrition, ease, environment, and taste) is what worked for George. Like George, you'll find this method to be simple, interesting, and doable in your own way.

» Read the label.

» Count the calories.

» Keep it NEET.

» Keep it simple.

» You decide. You choose. You win.

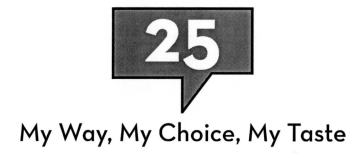

My Way, My Choice, My Taste

"Congratulations, George. That is a wonderful way for anyone to manage his or her eating habits in a healthful way," Ann almost shouted enthusiastically. "This way, everyone has a choice to design according to these parameters. You have shown me how important it is and also how to balance my eating habits to my satisfaction within these guidelines.

"In the past, I would be very strict with my prescribed diet and very unhappy and dissatisfied with a so-called healthy diet. At other times, I would go out of control and eat all the goodies and condemn myself for that.

"Instead of an all-or-none, win-or-lose scenario, you have suggested a balance that focuses on continuous efforts to make our eating habits better, without feeling guilty or condemning ourselves. You have shown how to face diet change as a new challenge every day, to make it better.

"Now I have an incentive to find my way to balance my nutrition and enjoy the pecan pie slice on one day and whatever else I may choose on another day—so long as I counter it with extra exercise or by cutting down caloric intake from ice cream, soft drinks, cookies, and so on.

"The PDDP will definitely help me to do that my way with my choice and with the taste I like.

"One request: Will you make a bulleted list of these points to keep on my kitchen wall as well as in my purse, so that I can review and reflect on those points every now and then to keep me on track? I want to do it my way. I like that idea very much." Ann gave a big, confident smile.

"Thank you, Ann, for your compliments and confidence. John has already prepared such a bullet list for you and others like you," George responded.

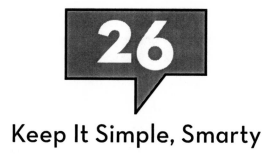

Keep It Simple, Smarty

It can be done.

—RONALD REAGAN

These are the secrets of George's success:

» Know what you want to do.

» Remember your goal.

» Read the label. Count the calories. Keep it NEET. Keep it simple.

» When it's about your own nutrition and health, find out:

» What inspires and motivates you to eat healthfully?

» Beware of the hidden barriers. Find them and defeat them.

» Take care of today. Don't worry about tomorrow. Tomorrow will take care of itself if you take care of today.

» Know that it's not easy.

» Learn to be humble; seek support.

» When you have doubts, remember Arjun. Ask questions.

» Find a mentor; be accountable.

» Get a map. Know where you're going and why you're going there.

» Know your companions. Who is going with you (calories, sugar, sodium, fats, fiber, etc.)?

» Go after your goals with all you've got, no matter what obstacles you encounter.

» Stay on the road you've selected for your healthy destination. The road will take you there when you continue to travel on that road toward your destination.

» Enjoy every step of the journey, the easy road as well as the strenuous road.

» Keep at it. Keep on track. Monitor your travel. Watch out for hazards on the road. If you fall off track, recognize that fact and get back on track without blaming or condemning yourself or getting angry at someone else who brings it to your attention.

» Make sure every day that the guy in the mirror is your true friend.

» Remember the little engine that could and say, *"Yes, I can, and yes, I will."*

Conclusion

Nothing will ever be attempted if all possible
objections must first be overcome.
–SAMUEL JOHNSON

As a physician practicing in rural West Virginia, I have had the opportunity to observe the tremendous gap between the available information regarding nutritious diet and the practice of such diet choices in the lives of many people. I have experienced difficulty in communicating the available information to patients, friends, and family. I have had the chance to visualize the difficulties to follow through and comply with the instructions. I have experienced and listened to many excuses, objections, reasons, and "special" individual barriers.

Many people feel that nothing bad can happen to them, no matter what they do to themselves. I was no exception. I'm not perfect, but I have learned to be on the path, which I have found to be simple, useful, and enjoyable, and I try to make it better every day. As everyone knows, there are more ways than one to eat a delicious and nutritious diet.

My mantra to defeat the barriers to healthful eating:

Read the label. Count the calories. Keep it NEET. Keep it simple.

Make the guy in the mirror your true friend and *you* do what you would want him to do.

It gives me great pleasure to share this experience with you, with the hope that it will enrich your life as much as it has mine. Thank you for giving me this opportunity. I hope you enjoyed the stories and found answers to some of your barriers. I hope we will meet again soon and hear more success stories from each one of you. Good-bye. Au revoir. Auf Wiedersehen. Until we meet again!

Additional Resources

Plans are worthless, but planning is everything.
—DWIGHT EISENHOWER

Additional Reading

Dietary Guidelines for Americans, 2010

Fit and Well: Core Concepts and Labs in Physical Fitness and Wellness, McGraw-Hill

Obesity Education Initiative Electronic Textbook

Williams' Basic Nutrition and Diet Therapy, 14th ed. Elsevier Mosby

Resources

www.eatright.org

www.acsm.org

www.cdc.gov

www.fda.gov

www.nutrition.gov

www.calorieking.com

www.dashdiet.org

www.choosemyplate.gov

www.DietaryGuidelines.gov

www.google.com

Interesting Information

"You are what you eat." "Food is medicine, and medicine is food." Have you heard these expressions? Over the years, scientists have come to believe that a strong relationship exists between nutrition and health.

Being overweight or obese increases health risks from hypertension, heart disease, lipid disorders, type 2 diabetes, stroke, gall-bladder disease, osteoarthritis, sleep apnea and other respiratory problems, and certain cancers (endometrial, breast, and colon). Obesity is also associated with pregnancy complications, menstrual irregularities, hirsutism, stress incontinency and psychological disorders, body-image dissatisfaction, and higher morbidity.

The media delivers a powerful message that people should be thin and that to be fat is a sign of poor self-control. These negative attitudes toward the obese often result in discrimination in employment and housing opportunities, college acceptance, job earnings, opportunities for marriage, plane-ticket costs, health-insurance costs, and much more.

Obesity is a chronic disease, and successful treatment requires a lifelong commitment. Any excess calories (more than what the body uses on a daily basis) from any source (carbohydrates, fats, or proteins) are converted as storage fats, resulting in weight gain. The combination of a reduced-calorie diet and increased physical activity produces greater weight loss than diet or physical activity alone.

The following are the essential elements in human nutrition:

> » carbohydrates, proteins, fats (macronutrients)
> » vitamins, minerals (micronutrients)
> » water

The critical issue is not the relative proportion of the macronutrients in the diet, so long as there are no extremes. The critical issue is ensuring adequate intake of all the necessary nutrients, variety, distribution of sources, and Calorie balance, while keeping in mind taste and satiety.

As long as adequate amounts of essential fatty acids are supplied in the diet, the body is capable of manufacturing other fats and cholesterol as needed. Higher intake of saturated fatty acids and trans-fatty acids is associated with abnormalities in the lipid profile and cardiovascular diseases.

As long as adequate amounts of essential amino acids (building blocks of proteins) are supplied in the diet, the body is capable of manufacturing other proteins as needed. Essential amino acids are those amino acids for which synthesis by the body is inadequate to meet metabolic needs and thus must be supplied in the diet. More protein in the diet does not automatically result in building more muscle mass. Protein in the diet beyond what the body needs on a daily basis are converted into storage fat, and the excess nitrogenous waste products are cleared by the kidneys.

Carbohydrates have a bad reputation in the media, mainly because of our food choices. An increase in the intake of complex carbohydrates can help displace fatty foods from the diet. Foods rich in complex carbohydrates include vegetables, legumes, fruit, and whole-grain cereals, breads, and pastas. Simple carbohydrates (sugars) should come from food sources in which they are found naturally, such as fruit and milk, rather than from foods with added sugars, such as cakes, cookies, candies, soda, and fruit drinks.

Body-mass index (BMI)

BMI is the most commonly used tool today for simple and quick assessment in clinical practice. It describes weight relative to height. It's not perfect; it overestimates body fat in people who are very muscular and can underestimate body fat in people who have lost muscle mass (e.g., the elderly).

	Obesity Class	BMI
Underweight		< 18.5
Normal		**18.5 to 24.9**
Overweight		25 to 29.9
Obese	1	30 to 34.9
Obese	2	35 to 39.9
Extremely obese	3	40 or more

Overfat

This describes a normal BMI but abnormally high body fat according to body-composition tests, especially in the elderly and short individuals.

Waist circumference

The presence of excess fat in the abdomen is an independent predictor of risk factors and morbidity. Larger waist circumference indicates larger abdominal fat content.

High risk
Men > 102 cm (> 40 in.)
Women > 88 cm (> 35 in.)

Waist-to-hip ratio (WHR)

Hip proportion is measured at the widest portion of the buttocks; waist portion is measured at the midpoint between the lower margin of the last palpable rib and the top of the iliac crest. WHO STEPS states that abdominal obesity is defined as a WHR above 0.90 for males and above 0.85 for females.

Basal metabolic rate (BMR)

BMR is the number of calories that you need at rest for basic bodily functions, such as heart rate, breathing, digestion, and body temperature. BMR is responsible for 60 percent to 75 percent of our calorie needs. The calories required to digest food is called the thermic effect of food.

Total energy intake is the total number of calories you take in from carbohydrates, fats, and protein in your diet. The total energy expenditure is BMR + thermic effect + calories used for physical activity.

Diet

This describes the food and drink a person takes in day after day. It also refers to the amount of food consumed (e.g., 1,000-calorie diet) and to the kind of food consumed (e.g., vegetarian, diabetic, low-salt, Mediterranean, and so on). A normal or balanced diet is one that contains all the food elements needed to stay healthy.

Nutrition

This term refers to the process by which living organisms take in food and use it, and the science that explores foods and the way the body uses them. It also describes the balance between dietary intake and need.

Metabolism

This is the sum of all chemical changes that take place in the body, by means of which it maintains itself.

Calorie

A calorie is a measure of energy. In the study of nutrition, it refers to the manner in which the body makes use of the energy locked in the chemical bonding within food. Energy is released by the metabolism of food. The body needs energy for the processes of survival.

Among these processes are

» chemical reactions that accomplish synthesis and maintenance of body tissues;

» electrical conduction of nerve activity;

» production of heat to maintain body temperature; and

» mechanical work of muscle effort.

How many calories do you need on a daily basis?

To maintain steady weight, you need to take in as many calories as you burn daily. If you take in more calories than you use, the excess calories are stored as fat—and you gain weight. If you take in fewer calories than you need, your body uses its stores, and thus you lose weight.

What is the difference between calories (energy)
from fats, proteins, and carbohydrates?

None. Energy from any source is used as the fuel for bodily functions. A thousand calories from carbohydrates are equal to 1,000 calories from fats or proteins.

Calories (energy) derived from fats, carbohydrates, and proteins are the same, but the amount of energy (number of calories) in a fixed portion size of food is different. A bucket of apples has fewer calories than the same-sized bucket of cheese. And as you know, the building materials in apples are different than the building materials in cheese.

One gram of fat has nine kcal.

One gram of carbohydrates has four kcal.

One gram of proteins has four kcal.

One gram of alcohol has seven kcal.

Empty calories are those that lack fiber or any other nutrients, such as minerals and vitamins. The body uses empty calories in the same way it uses calories from other foods.

Do calories from sweets really tend to make you
fatter than calories from vegetables?

Yes, because sweets have higher concentration of calories (high caloric density). A specific amount of sweets contains more calories than the same amount of vegetables by weight or volume.

How many calories does an adult with average daily
activities need to maintain current weight?

About 1,500 to 2,000 calories. See ChooseMyPlate.gov for more guidance.

How many calories does it take to lose one pound of body fat?

One pound of body fat is equal to about 3,500 calories. Losing one pound requires burning 3,500 more calories than you take in. Walking one mile burns about a hundred calories. So you need to walk or run thirty-five miles to lose one pound of weight, which is very difficult for most people. Therefore, controlling the intake of energy (calories) is very important.

Does running one mile burn more calories
than walking one mile?

There's no significant difference. Both require about the same number of calories, but running one mile takes a much shorter amount of time.

Cholesterol

Cholesterol is a fatty substance found in the bloodstream. Your body manufactures all the cholesterol it needs to build important hormones and construct cells. Therefore, there's no dietary requirement for cholesterol. Too much cholesterol can cause plaque buildup in the arteries and restrict blood flow to the heart and other organs. Cholesterol intake should be limited. Bile is made in the liver; it is normally recycled. It is 70 percent cholesterol. Bile is needed for the emulsification of fats. Some medicines and foods, such as oatmeal, flax seeds and dietary fiber, remove bile from the gut and lower your cholesterol.

What is bad cholesterol?

Low-density lipoprotein (LDL) cholesterol is often referred to as "bad" cholesterol. An excess of LDL may deposit cholesterol on the walls of the arteries over time. These deposits may eventually clog arteries leading to the heart, which in turn can lead to a heart attack.

What is good cholesterol?

High-density lipoprotein (HDL) cholesterol is considered good for your body because it is thought to carry cholesterol away from the arteries and to the liver for elimination.

Fats

Fats are made of the same elements as carbohydrates—carbon, hydrogen, and oxygen. They are compounds of fatty acids and glycerol.

We have many different ways of classifying fatty acids: saturated versus unsaturated; essential versus nonessential; short-chain, medium-chain, and long-chain; omega-3, omega-6, and so on.

The functions of fat include energy storage, thermal insulation, insulation to protect vital organs from trauma, vitamin transfer, hunger suppression, the synthesis of many hormones, and brain development and function. Fats also add taste and texture to food. As long as adequate amounts of essential fatty acids are supplied in the diet, the body is capable of manufacturing other fats and cholesterol as needed.

It is not easy to reduce the fat content in food because fat contributes significantly to taste. However, eating foods that are high in fat, especially saturated fat, can raise the level of cholesterol in your blood, which is not good for you.

To reduce fat intake in your diet, do the following:

- » Bake, steam, boil, or broil foods instead of frying.
- » Use nonstick vegetable-oil cooking spray instead of butter or oil.
- » Remove the intake of high fat foods.
- » Use low-fat substitutes.

Saturated fats

These fats are usually solid at room temperature. Although they are most commonly found in animal products, saturated fats also occur naturally in such vegetable products as chocolate and coconut and in vegetable products that have been converted from a polyunsaturated fat to a saturated fat through hydrogenation (trans-fatty acids). Trans-fats are unsaturated vegetable oils that manufacturers hydrogenate to make solid so they can last longer. It's important to read food labels carefully. Although a label may correctly say "no cholesterol," the product may contain a high level of saturated fat. Higher intake of saturated fats and trans-fatty acids is associated with abnormalities in the lipid profile and cardiovascular diseases.

Monounsaturated and polyunsaturated fats

These fats are usually liquid at room temperature and are found primarily in vegetable products.

Essential fatty acids

The body needs these fatty acids for various reasons; because it can't manufacture enough of these fats on its own, you must get them from your diet. There are two of these: linoleic acid (an omega-6 fatty acid) and alpha-linolenic acid (an omega-3 fatty acid).

Sources of omega-6 fatty acids include meat, corn oil, safflower oil, sunflower oil, and canola oil. Sources of omega-3 fatty acids include cold-water fish, flaxseed oil, walnuts, dark green leafy vegetables, canola oil, tofu, and soybeans.

Most people consume much more omega-6 than omega-3, but proper balance is very important because of the pro-inflammatory and anti-inflammatory effects of these fatty acids. This balance can be accomplished by reducing your consumption of meats, dairy products, and refined foods while increasing your consumption of omega-3-rich foods such as cold-water fish, flaxseeds, walnuts, tofu, and dark green leafy vegetables.

Carbohydrates

Carbohydrates are made of the same elements as fats—carbon, hydrogen, and oxygen. They are our main energy source. They also maintain the body's store of quick energy reserves as glycogen. They are widely available. Carbohydrates have a bad reputation in the media mainly because of our food choices.

Carbohydrates exist in multiple forms, from simple to complex. Simple carbohydrates include monosaccharides and disaccharides (sugars). Complex carbohydrates include polysaccharides, consisting of twenty or more sugar units stuck together. An increase in the intake of complex carbohydrates can help displace fatty foods from the diet. Foods rich in complex carbohydrates include vegetables, legumes, fruit, and whole-grain cereals, breads, and pastas. Simple carbohydrates (sugars) should come from food sources in which they are found naturally, such as fruit and milk, rather than from foods with added sugars, such as cakes, cookies, candies, soda, and fruit drinks.

The Food and Nutrition Board has set the acceptable macronutrient distribution range for added sugars at 25 percent of total daily calories. But World Health Organization guidelines limit calories from added sugars to 10 percent of total daily caloric intake.

The glycemic index and glycemic load measure how quickly your blood sugar rises after ingesting a particular food. Oatmeal, whole grains, nontropical fruits, legumes, beans and peas, and minimally processed foods generally have a lower glycemic index, but the index is altered by many factors.

Fiber

Fiber is the indigestible fraction of food from plant sources.

Water-soluble fibers (gums, mucilages, pectins, and so on) include barley, rice, corn, oats, legumes, apples, and pears. Water-soluble fiber lowers LDL cholesterol, delays glucose absorption, and limits the rise of postprandial insulin levels.

Water-insoluble fibers (lignins, cellulose, and so on) include root and leafy vegetables, whole grains, cereals, bran, and cruciferous vegetables such as cabbage, broccoli, and Brussels sprouts. Water-insoluble fiber reduces constipation, diverticular disease, and colon cancer.

Both epidemiological studies and clinical trials have determined that a diet high in fiber may contribute to a reduced risk of various chronic diseases. The National Cancer Institute recommends consuming twenty to thirty grams of fiber per day.

Dietary fiber has several reported benefits:

- » laxation
- » reduction of cholesterol level
- » displacement of saturated fat and cholesterol from the diet
- » improvement of glycemic control among patients with type 2 diabetes
- » treatment and prevention of diverticulosis of the colon
- » reduction of colon-cancer risk
- » reduction in hunger sensation and therefore reduction in amount of food eaten

What are probiotics?

Probiotics are living organisms that, when administered in adequate amounts, confer a health benefit on the host. The most common probiotics are certain types of bacteria.

What are prebiotics?

Prebiotics are indigestible nutrients (fiber) in our diet that serve as food for the bacteria (probiotics) in our digestive tract.

Proteins

Proteins, like fats and carbohydrates, contain carbon, hydrogen, and oxygen. They are unique because they also contain nitrogen, along with sulfur and sometimes elements like phosphorus, iron, and cobalt. Proteins are complex nitrogenous compounds made up of amino acids in peptide linkages.

Proteins are important for building and repairing tissue and for building other important chemicals that make the body function— for example, immune cells and enzymes. They also help with acid-base balance and the transport of other substances in the blood. Mechanical proteins are found in muscles and are needed for muscular contractions. Proteins are also a source of energy, but proteins are not the primary source of energy. They are used for energy only when other energy sources are inadequate or cannot be used properly.

A normal adult needs 0.8 grams of protein per day per kilogram of ideal body weight, depending on your weight range, weight-management plan, and physical activity. The body needs a daily supply of amino acids to make new proteins. Your body can store fat, and you have a small ability to store carbohydrates in your muscles and liver, but you can't store protein. If you don't replenish protein on a daily basis, you lose protein from some part of your body. As long as adequate amounts of essential amino acids are supplied daily in the diet, the body is capable of manufacturing other proteins as needed. Essential amino acids are those amino acids for which synthesis by the body is inadequate to meet metabolic needs and thus must be supplied in the diet. With genetic code as a blueprint, protein is built from essential and nonessential amino acids in food. Complete proteins contain all the essential amino acids. They are mostly of animal origin or from soybeans or quinoa. Incomplete proteins are missing an essential amino acid or do not contain an adequate amount. These are mostly from plant sources. You can combine incomplete proteins to create a complete one.

Getting more protein in the diet does not automatically result in building more muscle mass. Proteins beyond what the body needs are converted into storage fat, and the excess nitrogenous waste products are cleared by the kidneys.

A diet high in animal protein provides adequate essential amino acids to ensure efficient protein synthesis. But such a preponderance of animal proteins is not necessary. A vegetarian diet can provide all the necessary proteins, especially if it includes milk and other dairy products. Most people ingest a mixture of foods in a meal, and when available in sufficient quantity the various proteins tend to complement or supplement one another by creating a mixture containing all the essential amino acids.

> » Carbohydrates
> » energy primary source
> » energy quick store (glycogen)
> » protect fat breakdown
> » bulk, fiber
> » Fats
> » secondary store, long term
> » essential nutrients and chemicals for tissue building
> » bring in vitamins
> » support, padding for internal organs
> » taste, texture, satiety
> » Proteins

- » tissue building and repair
- » chemical agents for regulatory functions
- » mechanical activity
- » energy provider of last resort

Vitamins

Vitamins are organic compounds that are essential in small amounts for control of metabolic processes; they cannot be synthesized by the body.

Are daily vitamin supplements necessary?

Only in certain special situations. For example, B12 (cyanocobalamin) supplements are suggested for elderly people on a vegetarian diet.

Minerals

Minerals are inorganic substances that the body needs in small amounts. The body needs seven major minerals (calcium, phosphorus, potassium, sulfur, sodium, chlorine, and magnesium) and fourteen trace minerals (iron, selenium, iodine, chromium, zinc, fluoride, copper, manganese, molybdenum, boron, silicon, vanadium, nickel, and strontium).

Diets high in protein and sodium can limit the bioavailability of calcium. Too little vitamin D can also affect calcium absorption.

Healthy adults should consume no more than 2,300 milligrams of sodium per day. Older individuals and those who have high blood pressure should aim to consume no more than 1,500 milligrams of sodium per day. Individual preference for salt varies, so by reducing the amount of sodium in your diet, your preference for salt will decrease. Use other flavorings to help with the taste. Remember, just because food doesn't taste salty does not mean that it is low in sodium. It is therefore *most* important to focus on food selection (eating more fresh and frozen food and fewer processed, sodium-laden foods).

Measurements

Measurements on the labels provide information regarding the amount of food, calories, nutrients, servings per container etc. But unfortunately, many different measuring ways are used to provide this information. Example: cubic centimeter (cc), cup, gram (g), hand-sized, fist-sized, large, medium, small, milliliter (ml), number of calories, number of items, ounce (oz.), by weight, ounce (oz.), by volume, pinch, pint, pound (lb.), quart, serving, size of a deck of cards, spoonful, tablespoon (tbsp.), teaspoon (tsp.).

Sometimes this can be very confusing. Therefore you must be very careful about the amount of food on your plate and the number of calories in that amount of food. To convert this information from the label to the food on the table definitely requires your full attention!

The List of Barriers

*Which of these barriers create obstacles
in **your** path to healthful eating?*

Don't know

- » why eating healthfully is important
- » what is eating healthfully
- » how to eat healthfully
- » whom to ask, what to believe
- » what the benefits of healthful eating are
- » what consequences do we have to face if we neglect the problem of obesity
- » whom to trust (TV, books, speakers, advertisements) = confusion and ignorance
- » about nutrition and need
- » about proper diet
- » about body functions, health, and diseases
- » about cooking processes, ingredients, and cooking skills
- » about the right questions to ask

Don't want to know

» fear of finding out (avoidance = knowingly turning a deaf ear and blind eye)

» fear of needing to be responsible (out of sight, out of mind)

» fear of failure ("I can't do it, so why try?")

» fear of public opinion ("What will they say if I fail?")

» wishful thinking, overconfidence, carelessness, or foolishness ("It will go away; it can't happen to me.")

» wrong set of beliefs ("I will pray it away.")

» feeling of inertia/apathy

» feeling of inability to tackle an additional problem

» fear of the cost (money or time)

» false feeling of freedom (carelessness, no rules, no inhibitions, no plans)

Want to know—but not really

» doing it for the wrong reasons (equating being slim with being pretty)

» selecting the wrong motivator or guide

» choosing the wrong method

» working hard but hardly working

» being stubborn and inflexible (and stupid or ignorant); thinking that you know but don't and thus working frantically on the wrong track; getting worried and angry about the results and about what "they" say and finding excuses to justify yourself

» not knowing the right questions to ask

Unable to know

- » naive
- » arrogant
- » unable to recognize warning signs
- » ignorant of "normal" bodily functions
- » disregard for warning signs

Know, but cannot implement

- » lack of inspiration, initiative, motivation, desire, drive, peace, focus, etc.
- » lack of willpower
- » lack of consistency
- » procrastination (by habit or nature)
- » inertia ("I'll start tomorrow.")
- » laziness ("I'm not ready today. What's the hurry? I have so many important things to do before I can get to this one.")
- » resistance to change
- » inability to take on one more problem (already have too many burdens)
- » lack of money
- » lack of time to learn and act
- » lack of self-discipline
- » wrong environment (self-discipline not possible)
- » lack of specific information, skills, tools, or teachers
- » lack of encouragement or support
- » ignorance of or disbelief in the benefits of planning
- » driven by the immediate pleasures of the sense organs
- » fear of change
- » fear of failure

» lack of faith in teacher, information source, or data

» cynicism ("So many times the data is proved wrong later, as with drug recalls.")

» lack of usable skills

» tendency to blame everything and everybody else for your failure

» lack of convincing reason to accept change

» complacency in current situation

» feelings of anger, guilt, or stress (and a habit of running for pleasure to comfort foods)

» feelings of arrogance ("I've always done it like this.")

Know but will not implement; will not use the information; do not want to do it (self-destructive)

» lack of confidence

» poor self-image

» feelings of hopelessness

» failure in previous attempts

» discouragement

» inertia or lack of focus, urge, and priorities ("I'll start tomorrow, after my vacation, after Christmas …")

» dislike of hard work and pain

» "you only live once" attitude

» complacency ("I'm all right; it won't happen to me.")

» willingness to blame failure on someone or something else

» refusal to give up "only enjoyment," such as ice cream, cake, pie, cookies, soft drink, snacks, or alcohol

» inability to get into the mind-set to accept new information (looking for reasons to justify old behavior)

» misplaced, skewed ideas ("I have a right to do what I want. My family has always lived this way. I like to live on the edge. God will take care of me.")

» ignorance of or refusal to accept information about costs and benefits

Specific disease conditions e.g. thyroid disorder

» not taking necessary medications

» adverse effect of some medications

» experiencing a disease state (physical or emotional)

Author Information

After graduating from medical school in Bombay, India, S. L. Bembalkar came to the United States for postgraduate medical education. After completing postgraduate training in Louisville, Chicago, and Denver, he joined a multispecialty group practice in Beckley, West Virginia, in 1973. He is married and has one son. He is happily working as a board-certified internist with AccessHealth, a multiphysician group in Beckley, West Virginia. He is a member of the American Medical Association, and the Obesity Society.

CPSIA information can be obtained at www.ICGtesting.com
Printed in the USA
BVOW03s1851110814

362475BV00001B/7/P

9 781480 808508